Activities for Older People

Acquisitions editor: Heidi Allen
Development editor: Zoe Youd
Production controller: Chris Jarvis
Desk editor: Jane Campbell
Cover designer: Alan Studholme

Activities for Older People

A Practical Workbook of Art and Craft Projects

Brian W. Banks

WITHDRAWN

BUTTERWORTH
HEINEMANN

OXFORD AUCKLAND BOSTON JOHANNESBURG MELBOURNE NEW DELHI

Butterworth-Heinemann
Linacre House, Jordan Hill, Oxford OX2 8DP
225 Wildwood Avenue, Woburn, MA 01801-2041
A division of Reed Educational and Professional Publishing Ltd

ℛ A member of the Reed Elsevier plc group

First published 2000

British Library Cataloguing in Publication Data
A catalogue record for this book is available from the British Library

Library of Congress Cataloging in Publication Data
A catalog record for this book is available from the Library of
Congress

ISBN 0 7506 4741 8

Typeset in Bauhaus and Univers by David Gregson Associates,
Beccles, Suffolk
Printed and bound in Great Britain by Martins the Printers,
Berwick upon Tweed

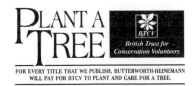

Contents

Contents

Chapter 3
Working with paper   63

Chapter 4
Modelling with clay, Plasticine and
salt dough   92

Contents vii

Chapter 5
Weaving 115

Chapter 6
Stencilling and block printing 135

Chapter 7
Glass and silk painting 153

Contents

Contents

Preface

At the time of writing this book my involvement in the visual arts has spanned more than a quarter of a century, most of which has been spent teaching in further education and recreational studies in Canada. These experiences have brought me into contact with people of different ages, from many walks of life, many of whom were in their retirement years. My instructional work also involved setting up art programmes in a geriatric ward, and a workshop in a home caring for patients with Alzheimer's disease.

On my return to England in 1996 I was drawn to working with people in care, and found that those in this situation were not given the opportunity to do very much other than play games of cards or watch television; most, unfortunately, slept the days away. Knowing that the visual arts are very stimulating, I decided to find a position that would allow me to organise my own activity programme with older people. My quest was soon answered, and such a position was offered to me in November 1997. It involved arranging activities in a residential care home, the majority of whose residents suffer from dementia.

It is common knowledge that one can still learn new skills and enjoy new experiences well into old age. Those who grow old but involve themselves in some activity stay healthier and enjoy life much more than those who don't.

As I have been involved with many forms of the arts, I was able to introduce the residents to watercolour painting, weaving, pottery, modelling and many other forms of craft work.

I could see that my work at the care home brought several of the residents out of their armchairs, from a state of lethargy, and into an environment where they could explore the world of creativity, even if it was to a limited degree. It also gave them the opportunity to observe several different art and craft ventures in progress, a first-time experience for most. The residents were also conversing with one another about their childhood days and families, which was a real bonus.

Over the many years I have been teaching I had often thought about writing an instructional book that covered drawing and painting, but could not find a direction for the content that was uniquely different from the hundreds of titles available.

In researching resource material for art and craft activities, I found that instructional books available from the libraries, bookshops and art shops tended to be very complex and usually focused on one topic only. The other alternative was to use children's colouring books, which I felt would be very degrading for older people.

As I found, one has to be very careful not assign projects and exercises that are too menial or childish or, on the other hand, too difficult. My experience in the residential home gave me the inspiration to start compiling projects that I had used successfully. I felt it was time that I started to assemble these projects into a book. An important consideration was to include activities that would be interesting but not too complex. Older people could then use the information and work through some creative projects by themselves, or be helped if necessary. The projects I have selected for the book are therefore not too complex but are still interesting and, above all, stimulating.

Some of the projects do require some artistic experience, most do not; however, in chapter 1 have included a section that will help the reader gain those necessary skills. I have always advocated that art skills can be learnt by anyone willing to spend a little time on the subject, no matter what their age. By learning these few basic artistic principles and techniques the reader will be able to work more easily on those particular projects or help others enjoy, and be stimulated by, them.

The projects can either be worked through by the reader or can be used to work alongside another person or people. If the reader is going to work with or help another person, I would suggest that he or she acquaint themselves with some of the procedures first, especially if these procedures have not been attempted before. The chapter on drawing and painting is one that the reader would be well advised to study before offering any instruction. Although quite technical, it gives one an insight into basic drawing and painting procedures.

Most of the projects in the book have been used successfully by me, and with older people. I have had to simplify some of the processes for them. Included, where appropriate, are suggestions that would suit a person with more ability. I would invite those undertaking this type of work to experiment and enlarge on these ideas.

There are several different aspects of art and craft work for the reader to drawn upon. When choosing an activity, I would suggest that you try a range of projects with each person, to find which of them he or she does best with. When working with men I have found it necessary to give them images or designs that they can better relate to, such as wildlife, buildings or landscapes: a good policy is to ask for their input before giving them something to work on.

I have also included a chapter on games and quizzes, as I have found activities in a group setting to be very stimulating for the residents. Several members of the group that I work with do not have a long attention span, so a group activity can be used to regain someone's attention and interest. These activities can also be used to break the ice with a new group.

If you are working in a care home or hospital environment, you might find that a group game is popular. Some of the patients or residents may not even wish to participate in an arts and craft programme, but they may well enjoy a quiz from time to time. I run a weekly quiz, and have enough residents to form a team game; they play for the honour of the winning team being awarded the house trophy. The change that these people go through, from their usual impassive condition to very enthusiastically voicing answers to questions at quiz time is absolutely amazing.

Brian W. Banks

Acknowledgements

I started writing this book about 10 years ago on odd scraps of paper and envelopes. After many twists and turns in my life, those notes and many other experiences and ideas have culminated in a manuscript. It has taken a while, but the journey was evidently necessary. This book would not have got to this stage without the help and guidance of many people. I would therefore like to thank the following: the Canadian friends and colleagues who supported and encouraged me over the years during my time in Canada as an art educator; Joan Smallwood, who gave me a completely free hand to work with the residents of The Lodge Residential Care Home; B & M Care, who allowed me to take and use photographs of the residents working on projects; and Sylvia West, who gave me some excellent ideas for the weaving projects. My heartfelt thanks go to the residents, past and present. Their eager participation gave me the motivation to write this book. And lastly, but by no means least, Betsy Evans, my dear friend and supporter throughout, who diligently read, suggested amendments, re-read, corrected and edited the text in progress. I thank you all.

Introduction

Research has shown that there is significant improvement in a person's wellbeing when they become involved in an enjoyable activity. I can certainly testify to this, as there was always a very positive change in the many people who came to my recreational art classes. This book will hopefully encourage the reader, or those caring for older people, to use the art and craft projects to stimulate and improve their quality of life.

For those who have not had much experience in the fine arts, I have included in chapter 1 a section on developing artistic skills. This will help the reader become more proficient in designing, drawing and painting. I have also included information and techniques on the various media used in the projects at the beginning of each section. At the end of the book you will find a number of pages of patterns; they are to be used in the appropriate project. Some of the patterns are full size so they can be traced and simply transferred. If you wish to use a design several times I would suggest that you make a template using heavy card.

I use art and craft projects in my day-to-day work with older people, all of whom have dementia of some severity. There is no doubt that their quality of life has improved greatly since I started working with them in this way. This book can be used as a guide for those in a caring situation to introduce art and craft projects to patients, clients, family or friends in their care. The projects and activities are specifically designed for older people and those with cognitive difficulties. No experience is necessary to teach these projects, as helpful advice and instructions are included in each chapter. There is, however, a need for some special materials. Some will be found around the home, others are available from your local art supply shop or from the mail order companies listed at the end of the book. I have used most of the projects explained in the book with older people, all of whom were in their seventies, eighties or nineties. A selection of their paintings was even entered into a competition, with great success. This was not so much to win prizes as for the residents to see their own work framed and hanging on a wall, which was a great confidence booster.

If you are in a position to help others, and are hopefully stimulated by the projects throughout this book to delve further, do enjoy yourself! Don't worry if some projects do not turn out as well as you had hoped. Enjoy the moment. If you are enjoying it yourself, there is a good chance that the people with whom you are working will too!

One of the important factors that I have been aware of, during my many years of teaching, is to accept everyone on an equal footing, and to give each person the same concentrated attention.

If the reader is working in a residential home or with a large group of people, I suggest that only three or four people attend a craft activity session at one time. This will prevent your being overwhelmed with questions and cries for help. A small group also allows for more individual attention, which is especially important with new group members and when the instructor is new to the group. I certainly do not expect everyone in the group to be doing the same activity. I have several different activities ready to start during a session, just in case someone needs a change or finishes a particular project quickly. I would also suggest keeping the length of each session reasonable; each person has a different attention span, and of course older people tire quickly. Having said that, I have had people who have wanted to stay longer than the usual two-hour session.

Treating each person individually, and giving them time to gain confidence and trust in me has been the main reason for the success of my activities pro-gramme. Everyone has such different capabilities and interests that I make a point of discussing their life experiences with them on an individual basis. As these capabilities and interests vary so widely, intro-ducing them to a series of projects and art media that require different skills is a good way to introduce them to the activities programme. However, I have found that the generation of people with whom I work have never experienced, or even seen, some of the activities I have introduced to them. I therefore try not to overwhelm them with too many things. Once they have more confidence and become more relaxed with me, I can introduce other media and activities. For those who are in need of help and support on a one-to-one basis, I arrange a time when they can have my undivided attention.

I try to evaluate each person's capabilities and interests as soon as possible. It gives me a guide as to what activity or medium they would enjoy. I do this by asking them to draw a picture from memory, or to copy a simple sketch or photo and then colour it, either with felt-tipped pens or paint. Modelling with Plasticine is also another excellent starting point. It is important that I do not give them some-thing either too simple or too difficult, both of which, I feel, would have a negative effect. So this introduc-tory period is time well spent.

One of the biggest considerations if you are working with people with dementia is memory loss. This can, of course, vary from person to person and can be somewhat frustrating. Sometimes, hours or minutes after completing a project, the creator does not recognise it as being his or her work. Before leaving a session, each person has to identify their work with their name. On many occasions I have had to explain, sometimes at great length, that it is indeed the person's work. Then he or she has always been absolutely delighted.

In my teaching method I have adopted a simple technique of using praise wherever possible. I avoid criticism and never belittle participants. Praise, and showing others the good points in a piece of work, is one of the best stimulants. It is especially important when working with people who have low self-esteem. I have found this often to be the case with older people and those with dementia. Giving praise and encouragement, without being patronising, does, I feel, build a lot of confidence.

I usually start participants off with a simple project, sometimes asking for their help on something that I have started. This is an excellent way to get them involved without overwhelming them. Unfortunately, trying to teach people with dementia can be exhausting, as instructions have to be continuously repeated. Each new session that they come to is the same as their first, with the simplest tasks sometimes having to be shown repeatedly. This, unfortunately, is their reality, so patience has to be exercised, and instructions have to be explained again.

I run a morning and an afternoon programme, and often a person asks if he or she can come to the afternoon session, completely forgetting that they had been to the morning session. Others just like to come to every session.

It is important that each person who takes part in my activities programme experiences and enjoys the process of working on a project. I do not expect great works of art, so I do not present standards that are hard for them to meet.

Many times I have been pleasantly surprised by the way some of the members get completely engrossed in a piece with just a little direction. One such person comes to mind. During her daily routine she is constantly anxious and agitated. As soon as she joins a session, usually a painting project, she becomes totally relaxed and will spend the whole session, which may last up to two hours, caressing the brush over the paper. The result is a painting of abstract qualities with layer upon layer of paint sometimes concentrated in only one area, but none-the-less a unique piece of work. She leaves the session totally relaxed and very grateful for the time that I have spent with her.

As my main purpose at the home is to improve the residents' quality of life, I try give to give them enjoyable tasks and projects. As they work on a piece, I usually ask if they have done anything like this work before. Often group members will recall their childhood days at their school's art classes, even remembering the teacher's name or sometimes a school friend. I find this to be a wonderful opportunity to open up a discussion, and often the other members will join in the conversation.

As with all of the residents' work, I do not analyse their finished projects. A rather humorous conversation with one of the members comes to mind, which typifies what a wonderful innocent humour they have. The woman in question worked in a very abstract style but tended to lose direction sometimes; with a little help she would get back on track and off she would go again. The project in this particular instance was to produce paper butterflies, which were to be strung together with others to form a series of mobiles. She progressed very well, using felt-tipped pens and colours of her choice, and completed the first side, filling in the design with tiny circles. I had not seen her colour like this before. I explained that as the butterflies were to be mobiles the other side had to be coloured as well. As she started on the second side I noticed that she had changed her colouring technique, and, instead of tiny circles, her strokes were much bolder and larger. This, I thought, was very interesting, and I felt that I could learn something from the total contrast in colouring technique. She had, by now, almost finished the side, so I decided to ask her why she was using such different strokes with her felt-tipped pen. Without hesitation, she drew close to my ear, and asked me not to mention what she was about to say to anyone in the group. By this time

I was getting very curious and thought that I was to be privy to something really important. Well, she said, I'm trying to finish this side quickly because I want to go for a wee!

As I mentioned earlier, I want every member who comes to an activities session to experience the process of working, and not so much to have a technically accurate finished piece. When the project for the session involves painting, I usually sketch out something, just to give the member an idea of how a subject could look. From there, I let each individual go her or his own way. This is so important, as older people are not too concerned about being aspiring artists or creating something that is acceptable to others; neither do they have inhibitions about the use of colour, so I let them choose their colour schemes and make changes to the original design if they so wish. I find it really exciting and rewarding to observe the process that they go through and the work that these wonderful people create. The finished product may be nothing like my original sketch, it may even be a total discord of colours, but it really does not matter, as their work is always individual and unique. They will no doubt ask your advice and even want you to help a little. Use your judgement in this matter; stress that you would rather that they do the work, as you want it to be their work and not yours. Give advice of course, but do not criticize. Criticism is neither necessary nor beneficial.

I find that the sessions do not have to be too structured. If someone is getting restless or bored, a change of activity can help. I also use games and songs in my programme. This is a useful way to give them a change of focus or to 'break the ice' if this type of activity programme is a new venture for them.

The majority of the photographs throughout the book are of work produced by older people with dementia. The photographs give an indication of what can be achieved with a little guidance and a lot of patience. It has given me the realization that with the selective use of activities such as art and craft work, games and quizzes, the many people in a care home setting or confined in some way, can definitely be given an improvement in their quality of life.

Chapter 1

Creating a space and working with older people

Creating a space

To get the best results from the activities I have included in this book, I recommend that a separate room is made available or a small area is set aside. However, if this is not possible, the activities can be accomplished on a trolley, table or tray.

The types of art and craft activities I have included require a flat working surface, somewhere to store art materials and completed work, as well as a water source and a clean-up sink.

Good light is very important. For those with poor eyesight a table lamp is helpful; it should be placed so that no shadow is cast over the work. I suggest sitting at the same level as the participant to give good eye contact. It will also facilitate working along with the person if necessary. Have available a good variety of music to create a relaxing atmosphere; check with the participants for their preferred music. Light classical music and singalong tunes are usually enjoyed by everyone. If you record music onto 90-minute cassette tapes or use a CD player this will give you a reasonable length of playing time before you have to attend to the music system. If music cannot be recorded or played, a radio station playing this type of music can usually be found on your local FM band.

If a separate room is available, the completed colouring and painting work can be attached to the walls with 'Blu-Tack' or another non-marking adhesive product. Completed work can also be framed and hung. Whatever the displaying approach, it will make the room or space into a special environment that the participants will recognize as their own and, above all, one that they have helped to create. In the room I use, I have hung dozens of mobiles, each having many sequins attached, which sparkle with the slightest movement. On the windows are hung many glass paintings, all created at various activity sessions. On sunny days coloured light pours through giving the room a wonderful ambience. The walls are full of work made by residents who attend the activity sessions, and also by those who have died. It always surprises me that even those residents with acute memory loss remember that they've been in the activities room before.

I always ensure that the participants' names are on their work; this will help if a piece has to be worked on at a later date. It is even more important to have a name displayed when working with a person with memory loss; it takes only a few minutes after completing a project for it not to be recognized as theirs.

When working on art and craft projects, the size of a group is very important. It has been my experience that one gets much better results from working with a small group of three or four people for an hour than working with eight or more for a two-hour session. In a large group one cannot give adequate individual attention and it can be overwhelming when several of the members require help at once.

Reminiscent discussion is something that I like to encourage, even while working on a project. It can be most enjoyable for everyone in the group as the event can be shared with pleasure – another good reason for a small group.

If people are a little reluctant to join in with the group, I have found it beneficial to work with them on an individual basis. It is a very good opportunity to find out more about the person. You may even find it worthwhile not to involve them in any activity but to just have a casual chat with them for a session or two. If a person is reluctant to get involved with an activity, try starting a project yourself. A little way through the work you might ask for the person's help; then the involvement may begin quite naturally. Try other projects and find one that might be of more interest. I feel that if the person is observing, they are, to a certain extent, involved in the project. I recall one occasion while working in a care home. One particular woman, in her late eighties, refused to involve herself in a project for several sessions. She was always very pleasant but would not get involved other than as an onlooker. Eventually, she became more interested in participating, and took the plunge. A little patience is usually rewarded later with the person happily engaged in a project. One thing I have learned over the many years I have taught recreational subjects is that people are not interested in tackling anything that might be too difficult for them. It may also be the case that the person is just not interested in a craft activity. He or she may show more interest in a board game or quiz; several are suggested later in chapter 9 on games.

Each person's attention span varies, as well as the individual's physical stamina. This is very important to take into account when setting projects. As I mentioned earlier, a small group will enable you to suit different projects to individual requirements, and still allow you to give each person your attention.

Older people are set in their ways, they do not like big changes or doing something that they feel uncertain about or that makes them feel silly. One of the biggest tasks when giving instruction and trying to stimulate older people is to give them confidence and make them feel they are doing something worthwhile. You will probably find that they really enjoy colouring a predrawn image, especially if it is made into a special card, say, for a great grandchild. When choosing images to be coloured, I would not recommend children's colouring books; I find that the images are too childish. Also, as the images are usually printed with a thick outline, it does not give the colourer the opportunity to detour from the line,

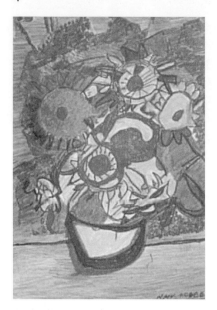

something that I strongly encourage. The final coloured image becomes unique. I would encourage everyone involved in this type of work to create his or her own designs, perhaps with the help of the person you are assisting. This approach will get them involved from the very beginning, even if you do the preparatory work. The process of creating a line drawing for colouring is quite simple and is outlined in chapter 2, projects 1 and 2.

The following is a list of recommendations I consider important when working with older people.

- Praise
- Listen
- Promote a discussion
- Make eye contact
- Show rather than tell
- Keep your expectations realistic

I would like to enlarge on the previous points as they are worthy of expansion.

Praise

It is difficult at times not to be condescending, especially when teaching older people. They need to be encouraged and praised, especially when involved in something completely new to them, which may be the case when working on the projects in this book. As I work with a group of people, it is a good opportunity to show and discuss each individual's work with the group. I usually draw their attention to the good parts in a piece, no matter how small. If there are areas that could be improved upon, it is important to discuss these as well. I do not criticize the work, as that would have a negative effect; instead, I suggest ways that might improve it. The other members of the group are always supportive and encouraging. This approach gives the originator of the work a good feeling and shows that others besides me are interested in their work. This same approach can be used when working with a single person. Showing their work to a relative or friend can be just as encouraging. I have heard many sad stories from people who have been totally discouraged by instructors who have negatively criticized their work. I have adopted the policy not to criticize, but rather to suggest changes that might improve the piece, always adding that it is from 'my point of view'.

Listen

Everyone needs to be listened to and older people are no exception. It is important to give them time to state what is really on their minds. We usually want to join in with our own viewpoints far too soon. I have found this especially true when talking with older people. They do tend to talk rather slowly and take longer to get to the point. So I allow them to take their time and make sure that they keep to the topic. It does prove difficult at times, especially when talking to people with dementia as they can have difficulty conversing. However, persevering and really listening to them can give an insight into their characters, their likes and dislikes and their opinions. This knowledge is invaluable, especially when developing an activity for a person. I am very much aware that a person needs to have confidence and trust in an instructor well before starting any activity. Listening and discussing their concerns helps them gain this confidence. Once I have their confidence, I have found that they become involved in an activity more quickly. As I have mentioned, I work in a residential care home. New residents are often confused and very upset in being placed in such a home, and take some time to settle in. Involving them as early as possible in something creative, or in a group activity that is fun, helps enormously with this transition.

Promote a discussion

If you have the opportunity to work with a group of older people, promoting a discussion is usually not too difficult. I have found that they are eager to discuss their family life and past experiences. It is unfortunate that those with dementia or with short-term memory loss do not remember such conversations from one day to the next. But because they can recall many things from their past and enjoy conversing on such topics, even though much repeated, it is good to let them talk openly. I have often observed someone who has hitherto been quite lethargic spring to life in such conversations.

It has been my observation that a good majority of care homes have lovely lounges, with the latest television installed in one corner of the room and comfortable armchairs set around the periphery. With most of the occupants asleep, conversation is usually minimal.

If a separate activities room is not available, I suggest a few chairs be drawn into a circle in a corner of the lounge. Turn the television volume down or off, and have some light music playing instead. I have a ready-made list of topics to discuss, just in case it proves difficult to get a discussion started. There are literally hundreds of topics that one could choose, such as school days, families, hobbies, sports, cooking, books, films, funniest events and so on. I try to keep to one topic, but having said that, being prepared for the unexpected is a necessity. I have instigated many discussions starting with a particular topic only to find the conversation wandering off track after only a few minutes. Actually, I have come to the conclusion that this is not a bad thing as it usually leads to a more interesting and spontaneous discussion from all the group members. The important thing is to involve everyone in the group. A person who is rather reserved, and doesn't say too much, often has a good deal to say when encouraged to get involved. This can be done by finding a topic that he or she likes or by asking a specific question about his or her past.

Several of our group discussions have led to heated arguments, especially when there is a personality clash in the group. This can be a little disturbing at first. The waving of arms and exchanging of heated remarks is not usually associated with people of 80 and 90 years of age. Usually they respond to a change in topic, and we get the discussion on track again. If there is a personality clash, this could lead to a discussion on such a topic. If it continues to be a problem, I find a plausible excuse to have one of them leave the group. The problem can then be discussed on an individual basis later. Discussing the problem with both people like this has often resulted in them becoming good friends later.

Make eye contact

This point seems obvious, but it is sometimes overlooked. I make it a point to maintain eye contact when I am instructing at any level. I feel that it gives the person an assurance that I am really working with them and am focused on their needs. If I am working on a project in a group, I endeavour to work with each person individually. This really helps me to see if they have fully understood what is required of them. When circumstances permit, it is preferable to position oneself at the same level as the participant.

Show rather than tell

When getting a group or a person involved in an activity, try starting with something quite simple and explain the procedure with a demonstration. This will give the participant(s) the opportunity to ask questions. By keeping the activity as simple as possible, they can be encouraged to try their hand. A person's capabilities can also be monitored more easily once he or she starts an activity. If people are reluctant to become involved in an activity, one has to be a little devious sometimes to get them interested. When working with Plasticine, clay or dough, I have formed a small piece of the substance into a ball and rolled it to the reluctant person. Usually they will stop it rolling onto the floor; I then ask them to roll it back to me – which they usually do! I keep up this process for a while, and try turning it into an amusing game. I might ask if they can squeeze the ball flat or make a sausage out of it when they pick it up again. Once they get to this stage, it is just a matter of slowly building their confidence and encouraging them to do more.

One particular woman has been coming to our group for 18 months and she is still a little timid about starting a project. The approach just described works every time. Knowing that she is very meticulous and likes everything tidy, I show her a colouring design that she might like to do. She usually says that it is far too difficult for her. If she shows an interest, I start to colour a small area, but purposely do not finish it or do not colour it very neatly. Invariably the woman concerned suggests that it would look better if I finished it properly. I then ask her to show me, at which point she gets completely involved, and happily carries on to finish the whole design.

Keep your expectations realistic

Some days, after working all day on a project or activity, I have felt that my accomplishments have been quite minimal and that I could have done much better. These days can be quite depressing, but usually when I weigh everything up, it has been because I expected too much from the people or individual with whom I have been working. If this happens to you, my advice is to do as I do, and lower your expectations.

Many of the projects throughout the book could have been shown with more complex designs or a more involved process. From my experience, working with older people, and especially those with dementia, I have found that they grasp procedures better when projects are simplified. The projects included in this book are starting points, and can be elaborated upon quite easily if you wish. If you do decide to make the projects more complex, I suggest that you measure the person's response first, using a simple project. People with dementia become confused easily. If they are given something to do with which they have difficulty they are apt to feel apprehensive and insecure. This can quickly lead to disinterest, and they may even want to leave. So, do monitor this carefully. Many residents with whom I work need to have instructions repeated at every session, and sometimes again after they have been to the toilet or have had a cup of tea. They have often totally forgotten what they were doing before the break. It is a good idea to keep a diary and record the person's responses and capabilities. The capabilities of older people, and especially those with short-term memory loss, can change from day to day.

Art materials

Art materials can be purchased at most stationery and art supplies shops, and a list of mail order companies is given at the end of this book.

Each project in the book is preceded by a materials list. The following is a description of some typical materials required for the projects throughout the book.

- Pencils: 2H, 2B, 4B
- Felt-tipped marker pens, mixed colour set
- Coloured pencils, mixed colour set
- Paper: white copier paper, watercolour paper, white card stock
- Tracing paper pad
- Carbon paper or transfer paper
- Scissors
- Brushes: for watercolours – short-handle synthetic fibres, round and 25 millimetres (1 inch) flat (one stroke)
- For painting with acrylics – hog-hair or synthetic fibres, round and flat
- Paints: watercolours, acrylics, glass paints, fabric paints

- Gutta, a resist for glass and fabric painting
- Ruler
- Pencil compass
- Palette or china saucers
- Glue stick, PVA glue
- Gummed paper
- Masking tape
- Clear adhesive tape

Support for stretching watercolour paper, 10-mm plywood, cut to suit size of paper. See watercolour paper stretching.

Pencils

A good stationery or art shop usually stocks a selection of pencils of varying grades.

Pencils are graded with a number and letter, the higher the number preceding an 'H' the harder the lead, the harder the lead and the lighter the pencil line. The higher the number preceding a 'B' the softer the lead and the softer the lead, the darker the pencil line. Pencils graded 2H and harder are useful for light tone work, and for pushing through an image onto another surface (this technique is explained later). Do not try to make the line or the shading darker by applying more pressure with this grade of pencil, it will only indent the paper. Hard lead pencil marks are also difficult to erase. Instead, use a softer pencil. When using softer pencils for shading, a slip-sheet under the hand will prevent the pencil graphite from being transferred to the hand. If you use 4B grade pencils or softer for dark shading, they will smudge easily. To help prevent this, an artist's spray fixative can be used.

Papers

Paper for general use

Paper is available in many weights (thicknesses) and colours. White copier paper, bought in a package, is ideal for general drawing and colouring work. It is economical and suitable for pencil, felt-tipped pen, and coloured pencils. I would not recommend it for fine work, watercolour or acrylic painting; if any water-based paints are applied the paper will curl and buckle.

Drawing paper

Drawing paper or cartridge paper is recommended for better quality work. It is available in pads or sheets and in a variety of weights from 96 gsm (grams per square metre). Pads are easier to use and store and they are readily available at stationery and art shops. The lighter weight papers are economical and suitable for pencil, pastel and charcoal work. The heavier cartridge papers will take a light wash, but again the paper is apt to curl when using watercolours very wet. I have seen many drawing pads labelled 'suitable for watercolour painting'; in fact they are not worth purchasing for that application.

Watercolour paper

For those wishing to try the watercolour painting projects I recommend that you invest in some good watercolour paper. This type of paper is manufactured especially for painting with watercolours. It is available in pad or sheets in a variety of weights and usually in three finishes: HP, hot pressed, NOT, also referred to as medium, and rough.

Hot pressed is a smooth-surfaced paper and can be quite tricky for the beginner to work on. It is used mainly for delicate and detailed work, 'wet-in-wet' or large washes are difficult to control. Medium is the paper commonly used by many watercolourists and the one I recommend. It responds well to large washes wet-in-wet and is also suitable for fine detailed work.

Rough has a very textured surface, It takes a good deal of paint to cover the surface. Many artists use this paper when they wish to create a 'sparkle' to a painting. The brush can be skipped over the paper's surface leaving tiny light spots. It is ideal for bold work.

The lighter weights are cheapest, and I recommend that they be stretched before applying paint (directions on stretching procedure is detailed in the watercolour project section). The heavier weights are more expensive, but they can be painted on without stretching.

Paint

I suggest that water-based paints be used wherever possible, as cleaning up is so much easier and toxic solvents are not necessary. The mediums included in this category are: watercolour, gouache, tempera, acrylic and water-miscible oil paint. A point to remember is that the watercolour medium is transparent; all of the other mediums are relatively opaque when used at full strength. Therefore, opaque colours can be painted over other colours to make changes or hide errors.

There is a large selection of paints and varying qualities available at vastly different prices. This can be a little confusing if you are not familiar with fine arts materials. Very cheap paints are not worth purchasing, as they will have very little actual colour and a good deal of filler in them. They will lead to a lot of frustration, with the painter failing to get good colour intensity. The colours will not be permanent either. My advice is to purchase the best that your budget will allow. The better quality paints will go much further; they are more intense and have a higher degree of permanency. If the painting is framed properly, behind glass, and kept out of direct sunlight it will last indefinitely.

One does not require a huge selection of colours to create a good painting. Restrict the number of colours, to begin with at least. A selection of no more than four basic colours is enough to get started. Other colours one might want in a painting can usually be mixed from these quite successfully.

By limiting the palette to fewer colours, the completed painting will harmonize much better.

Paints are produced in cakes, tubes and jars. It is better to buy the colours individually rather than in sets. One can always add to the range when more experience is gained. Suggested colours are indicated before each project in the painting sections of the book.

Paint should always be mixed in a palette or dish before applying it to the working surface. When working with watercolours, I would recommend the use of white china dishes or a large dinner plate. Saucers work reasonably well but it is important to stir the pigment from time to time as watercolours tend to separate and settle in the bottom of the dish.

Brushes

Hundreds of different brushes of various shapes and sizes are available. It can be rather overwhelming to have to select one for a particular purpose. Basically, short-handled soft brushes are used for water-based pigments or very detailed work. Long-handled brushes are usually used for oils and acrylics or paintings that are being produced on an easel.

Good quality artists' brushes can be very expensive; they are also available in lower quality for quite a lot less money. Here again, one has to decide on their use and the budget available. The cheaper quality brushes will not have so much spring in them – when moistened with paint or water they tend to go floppy. Hairs of these brushes often dislodge and come out while painting, which can be very annoying. I would suggest that you get something between the very cheap and the expensive. There are some very good synthetic brushes available that will last for a good time. Watercolour brushes need to have a nice spring in them; control can be easily lost when painting with cheap floppy brushes. The assistant at your local art shop will usually be happy to show you a selection. Ask to try the brush in a little water to check for springiness. The fibres of a brush usually have size applied at the factory, so you can only feel the actual spring in the brush when the size has been washed out. I also like to check to see if the brush will come to a natural point. To do this, dip the brush in the water and tap the ferrule, the metal part, on your finger. When working with watercolours, a good wash brush is required for large areas. This is usually called a one stroke brush and should be a minimum of 25 mm (1 In). Make sure that it has a good carrying capacity. Some of the cheaper brands do not. Don't be tempted to use a household paint brush as it will not give the results that an artist's brush will.

Always ensure the brush you are purchasing is suitable for the intended application; ask if you are not sure.

Developing artistic skills

As several of the projects in this book require some degree of drawing and painting skill, the objectives in this section are to familiarize the reader with some of those skills. These learned skills can then be used to help others if you so wish. More importantly, once these basic principles are learned, you will be able to create designs and subject matter of your own that can be used in projects throughout the book.

Over the many years I have been involved in the arts the remarks that I have heard time and time again when suggesting that a person try painting or sketching are: 'I'll never be able to draw, I can't even draw a straight line,' and, 'I just do not have any artistic talent, you have to be born with it, don't you?' These clichés have been passed on from one generation to the next, and I fear are ingrained in most people, so that they do not even attempt anything artistic. It is my belief that anything can be learned, and that, as in music and the visual arts, some will do better and learn faster than others.

One can always learn just the basics and go on to more advanced levels later if one so desires.

If you are in a position to help others, you will no doubt encounter some resistance when trying to teach drawing or painting to the elderly. Many of them do not wish to learn new skills, especially drawing, as this does test one's perceptual ability. However, I did meet one 90 year old man in a nursing home who had wanted all his life to be able to draw and paint, but had never found the time. He welcomed the opportunity to be taught some of these skills. You might find that others are very happy just to colour pre-drawn designs. As I mentioned earlier, if the outline is not too defined they usually wander away from the initial design. This to me is more important than their keeping to my lines. In fact, I encourage them to change lines and to add colours of their own choosing, because they then become involved in creating something relating to their own reality. The process is also delightful to watch; the result is a piece of art conceived more by the residents than by me. It is far more important that the person working on a project enjoys the process of working it through, rather than worrying about creating a technically correct work of art.

It is helpful to create designs from reference material unless you are an accomplished artist; photographs that you have in your own collection are a good source of information, as are the many periodicals available. Magazines usually have good photographs that can give you an idea for a subject or composition. Friends or relatives of the people you are working with are usually happy to pass on old copies of these magazines. If they are not useful for reference material, they will certainly be of use for collage work – you can cut out the coloured photographs and file them away for later use.

I have found that older people, in particular, are very aware that drawing of any kind is difficult for them. I had a comment from an elderly man that brought this point home. His observation was that 'people didn't like getting involved in art activities because they are afraid of making fools of themselves'.

The section at the end of the book on patterns and designs include some line drawings that can be photocopied, or traced and transferred to another surface. The projects in chapter 2, explaining the process of 'squaring up' to enlarge or reduce an image, will enable you to work from other images you may have, whether they are photographs or outline drawings. I feel that these projects can be accomplished fairly easily by anyone with good tactile skills, but help may be required when measuring and making the grids. I have often demonstrated this 'squaring up' process to a group, finding that they just like to watch as the image appears.

I would recommend that if the reader is to teach the projects to others they should try the projects first.

Drawing and shading techniques

If you have not had much art instruction, the following techniques will help you to get better results with colouring and shading work. You will find this very useful if you wish to improve your own work and also when showing others.

When colouring or shading large areas, there is a tendency to scribble in the area as fast as possible. This, of course, is how we used to colour – just watch a young child. One has to learn to control this urge to fill an area like this quickly. By far the more interesting approach is to apply short strokes close together (see Figure 1.1). They should be about 10 mm ($\frac{3}{8}$ in) and should nearly touch. (I use even shorter strokes for small work.) If the lines are drawn straight, in the same direction, they will make a flat texture (Figure 1.1a, b and c). As a good deal of work is done with felt-tipped pens, you will find that using the cross-hatching techniques as shown in this figure is very useful, especially when wishing to obtain lighter and darker areas. Overlapping the

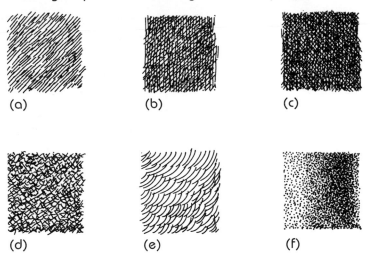

(a)   (b)   (c)

(d)   (e)   (f)

Figure 1.1

ends and beginnings of the lines is unavoidable, but this will make the overall effect more interesting. Another shading technique in Figure 1.1d shows how a dark tone can be built up by using a small X. By gradually overlapping and adding more Xs a variety of interesting tones can be created. The projects on shading in chapter 2 show this in more detail.

To give shape to a form the line can be curved (Figure 1.1e). If a gradual transition is required a dot (pointillism) instead of a line can be used to great effect (Figure 1.1f). The apple project in chapter 2 is a good example of pointillism.

When using pencils it is important to keep a constant pressure, and to keep the pencils sharp. Try various grades of pencil, from the soft 6B to the hard 3H to achieve different tones (values). You can also change the tone by using more or less pressure on a pencil.

With reference to Figure 1.2, one can see how a simple outline drawing can be transformed into a sketch that has some form and depth, just by adding directional and shading lines. The tree takes on a better form with the use of some curved lines, and darker areas become more interesting by using the cross-hatch technique.

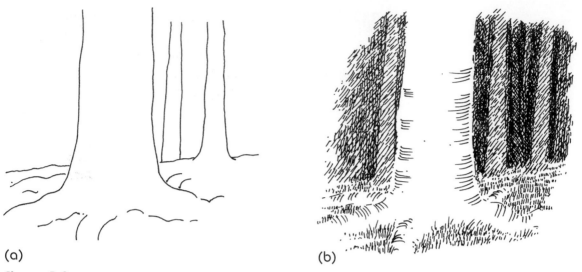

(a)   (b)

Figure 1.2

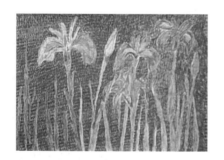

As I mentioned, coloured felt-tipped pens are often used in my activities programme; they are very easy for older people to hold and use. The shading techniques just described are ideal for this medium. Felt-tipped pens of different colours, cross-hatched over one another, give a unique vibrancy to the work. The textured background of the iris picture was obtained using the cross-hatch method. It took a lot of persuasion on my part to get the woman concerned to complete the work in such a manner. When finished she was highly delighted. The picture won a commendation at the over 60s art awards competition, run by the EAC (Elderly Accommodation Council).

Shading strokes can not only give form to a shape, they can also be used to emphasize a plane. A pathway is in a horizontal plane, a wall is in a vertical plane. Between these two planes lie many more angles. When drawing or painting paths, roadways, etc., the use of horizontal strokes will give the impression that the pathway is flat. Tilt the lines out of the horizontal and the pathway will also appear to tilt. Now try this on a wall or cliff. If the shading lines follow the vertical, the wall or cliff will look vertical. When drawing or painting a form that is not totally horizontal or vertical, this technique will help to establish its particular plane. Try this technique on smaller items that are around the home.

Grasses, twigs and branches can be given a natural look by lifting the pencil off the surface while the pencil is still in motion. When filling in large areas of grass keep the strokes going in one direction. The result will be more uniform.

Colouring pencils

Colouring pencils are another acceptable medium that older people enjoy. The pencils are easily controlled and as long as the person is able to hold a pencil, working with this medium should not be a problem. For those who have not had much experience with colour work, coloured pencils are an ideal way of experiencing colour and colour mixing. Some difficulty may be experienced with school grade colouring pencils, as they tend to be harder than the artist's grade. More pressure will have to be used to obtain rich colours, a point to consider for the elderly.

It is interesting to explore various working surfaces as different textures will result in a totally different appearance to the work. A rough surface will give a very grainy effect, while a smooth surface will give delicate shades, with almost a photographic appearance. Tinted surfaces can also expand one's creativity and should certainly be tried.

Pencils have to be kept sharp, especially when doing detailed work. To obtain various tones the pressure has to be altered – light pressure for light tones, heavier pressure for dark ones. Too much heavy pressure, with several layers of colour, can result in wax build up; this can show as an imperfection on the surface of the work. It can be removed with a tissue but care must be taken not to smudge the work. As with graphite pencil work, the finished work should be sprayed with fixative to prevent smudging.

Coloured pencils are transparent so colours can be mixed optically (laying one colour over another) in much the same way as watercolours when used as glazes. To maintain the freshness of a colour start with light colours and add darker ones on top. Lighter colours can be applied over darker ones to lighten them, but the brilliance is somewhat lost.

Because coloured pencils are similar to lead pencils, the stroke technique is very similar, but instead of just working in shades of grey, vibrant colours can be obtained by applying different colours on top of or next to previously applied colours. This colour mixing can be done in various ways. On a piece of paper shade a small area using yellow, cross-hatch (shade in different directions) over the top of this with light blue. The resulting colour will be a bright green. Apply different colours on top of the green and notice how they react. As there are dozens of different colours available the colour mixing combinations are endless.

A similar optical mixing can be obtained by using the pointillism and impressionism techniques. Dots or short lines of two different colours placed next to each other will result in a new third colour. Try a small study using three different colours. The pencils will have to be kept sharp, especially if using the pointillism technique. Impressionism is the technique of using complementary colours next to one another. Try the technique using short strokes and interweaving complementary colours together — red/green, blue/orange, yellow/purple, etc. You will see why Manet's first experiments with this painting technique influenced many other artists — Monet, Degas and Whistler, to name a few.

Once coloured pencils have been tried, you may want to try other mediums — water-soluble coloured pencils and pastels require similar application techniques. Unfortunately, chalk pastels are very dusty to work with, so I do not include them in my activities programme. Water-soluble coloured pencils are excellent and very easy to use. As water is used with this medium, I recommend watercolour paper be used. The colours can be applied first, and become soluble when water is applied. A brush is then used

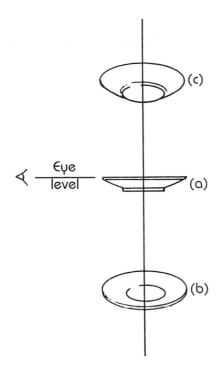

Figure 1.3

to blend and soften the colours. The resulting painting takes on the appearance of watercolours.
Another approach is to moisten the paper first and
then apply the colour, the colour softens on contact
with the paper. This gives a lovely loose drawing as
the lines bleed slightly.

Vases, pots and saucers

I have seen many well drawn and well painted
flowers but the vase or pot that they sit in has
often been very sad looking indeed. The following
is a very simple drawing technique whereby pots,
vases and the like can turn out looking something
like they should.

First I would like you to find a saucer. With reference to Figure 1.3, hold the saucer as shown (Figure
1.3a), with the rim of the saucer in line with your
eyes. You will notice that the rim appears as a horizontal line. Now lower the saucer a little, keeping it
level, and you start to see the shape of the saucer as
an ellipse. As you lower it further you will see that
the saucer becomes more circular (Figure 1.3b).
Place it on the floor and look into it; it has now
become almost a full circle. Bring it back to your
eye level, and raise it above your eye level a little;
again you will see that the shape of the saucer is
elliptical (Figure 1.3c). The higher it is above your
eye level, the more circular the shape becomes. What
you should notice in this exercise is that the diameter
of the saucer does not change, but the distance
between the closest and the farthest edge changes.
It gets larger as the saucer moves up or down from
the eye level. Saucers are generally at table height, so
place the saucer on a table, sit on a chair positioned
a little way away from the table, I suggest about
800 mm (32 in) away from the saucer. You will see
that the saucer is elliptical; try drawing it as you see
it.

If you are not happy with the results, try this approach. It's rather technical, but will give you an
introduction to some basic drawing procedure and

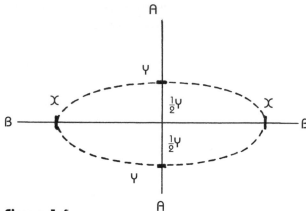

Figure 1.4

proportional drawing. With your 2H pencil draw a vertical line 'AA' (see Figure 1.4). Make sure it is vertical; use a ruler if you have to. We will refer to this line as the centre line of the saucer or its axis. Now draw a line, 'BB', horizontal to the vertical line 'AA'. When drawing ellipses in any plane or direction it is crucial that this line is always at 90 degrees to the axis line.

On the horizontal line 'BB' make a mark say 40 mm ($1\frac{1}{2}$ in) to the right of the vertical (XX) – it is not a crucial measurement. From this centre line make another mark on the horizontal line to the left, exactly the same distance from the centre line as the first mark. These two marks represent the diameter of the saucer. You now have to find the correct distance from the front edge to the back edge of the saucer. This is accomplished by a visual measurement (see Figure 1.5). If you find the procedure too complicated, just try to judge the distance. You could also try the principle of drawing size for size. This means that sizes from visual measurements are transferred directly to the working surface.

To do this measure distances with the point of a pencil and your thumb. Keep your hand fixed at arm's length when doing this. Transfer these measurements directly onto the paper. Try this procedure with other items around you. The finished drawing will be rather small, but it should give you an under-

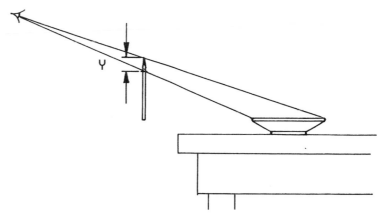

Figure 1.5

standing of the principle of proportions. Remember that to keep the drawing of the saucer symmetrical and level, always use the vertical and horizontal reference axis lines.

When checking measurements visually, make sure that your arm is fully extended and that the pencil is vertical and not tilted in any way. Close one eye and line up the tip of the pencil with the farthest edge of the saucer, adjust the tip of your thumb to line up with the front edge of the saucer. Now turn your hand horizontally, do not move your thumb, and measure as accurately as you can the number of times this distance (YY) can be divided into the diameter of the saucer. Keep your arm fully extended. If you are positioned about 800 mm (32 in) away from the saucer it will be about $2\frac{1}{2}$ times. Try to think of this not as a measurement but as a proportional amount. Make a note of this amount. Return to your drawing and divide the measurement that you have on line 'BB' into this proportional amount of $2\frac{1}{2}$. Use dividers or a compass if you have them. It can be done roughly with the pencil and thumb method. Transfer this distance to the vertical line 'AA'. Do make sure that this amount is centred on line 'BB', $\frac{1}{2}$YY (see Figure 1.4) This proportional amount is the distance from the front to the rear edge of the perspective saucer from your viewpoint. If you were to stand, the distance from the front to the rear edge will get much bigger. The diameter remains the same. It does not matter to what size the diameter is drawn, as long as the proportions are adhered to. The ellipse will always appear correct to the viewpoint (level) that you are viewing the saucer.

Carefully proceed to draw the ellipse. You should now have an accurate drawing of the saucer's elliptical shape. It is important that the ellipse be nicely curved at the saucer's width (the diameter), not too flat or too pointed, as shown by the dotted line in Figure 1.4. Now try the same technique with a flowerpot or vase or bottle. It is always best to draw a central vertical axis before you start drawing; this ensures that the object will be upright and not leaning. Try this little experiment. Gather together a number of plates and saucers of varying sizes. Put them one by one in the same location, each time you do this sit at the suggested distance and take the proportional measurement of the ellipse, i.e. the number of times 'YY' fits into 'XX'.

You will find that the measurement is the same for each different size.

We have studied circular objects in a vertical position, now let us look at cylindrical objects in a horizontal position. We shall use a glass tumbler for this exercise. Lie the tumbler on its side on the table in front of you, as in Figure 1.6. Sit at the table so that you can reach the tumbler easily. Place the tumbler so that the rim is directly in front of you. The rim will be seen as a straight vertical line, if it is positioned correctly. Imagine the tumbler with a centre line (axis). Now turn the tumbler so that you can start to look into it; the rim becomes an ellipse and gets wider as you pivot the tumbler. Study the sketches in Figure 1.6a, b and c; notice how the centre line 'AA' changes angle as the tumbler moves. The diameter of the tumbler 'BB' lies on an axis that is always 90 degrees to the centre line, no matter what the position of the tumbler. The proportion of the ellipse 'XX' to 'YY' can be measured in the same way as previously described.

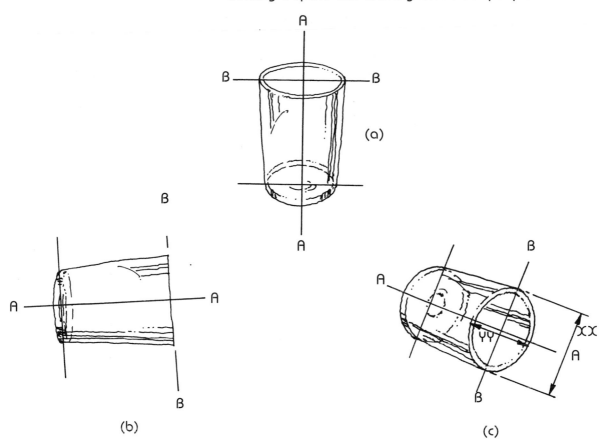

(a)

(b)

(c)

Figure 1.6

Design

There are many books devoted exclusively to design, so I will not get into this aspect of the arts too deeply. I feel it would be helpful to the reader to explain a few basic points. Every artist, no matter how experienced, would do well to rough out a design before proceeding with an artwork. If you have not had any art training, or it was some time ago, the following will help you and those you may be working with to produce better compositions. It will also give more awareness and appreciation when next looking at paintings, photographs, television or cinema photography. I often talk about the importance of design during a session, as some of the group members show a keen interest in the fundamentals.

The one underlining factor in all creative work is design. One only has to look around to see why design is so crucial. It is used in the creation of furniture, wallpaper, carpets, fabrics; virtually everything that is produced has had a designer involved.

When painting or drawing we should consider three basic linear forms: the horizontal, the vertical and the angle. The horizontal form gives a feeling of space, flowing left to right and right to left. A tranquil painting can be created using horizontal forms, say of a beach or looking across a lake. The vertical line is also used in painting. It is very useful in stopping the eye moving out of the picture area. Try a simple experiment: draw a small rectangle 50 mm × 75 mm (2 in × 3 in). With the longest measurement horizontal (in a landscape format) draw a horizontal line about a third down across the whole width, and another about two-thirds down, again across the whole width, at a slight angle to, say, represent a shoreline. It is apparent that the eye moves out of the frame very quickly. Now draw a vertical line close to the right-hand edge of the rectangle. It can go out of the top of the frame if you like. Notice it immediately stops this movement out of the picture to the right. Now place a mark on the water to represent a small boat; this will give the eye something to focus on. You now have the makings of a simple picture. Artists and photographers use this device frequently to hold and direct the viewer's attention.

The third line to consider is the angle. This line can be used to give direction, but also tension in a design, especially if it is straight and not curved. Try this procedure on a similar thumbnail sketch. Instead of using a vertical line, as before, tilt it an angle – first, towards the outer edge. You will find the eye moves out of the picture. Now erase this line and draw a similar line but move it a little off the vertical, towards the left, into the frame. The eye now moves towards the centre of the design. Increase the angle, and it becomes more forceful. If this line represents a tree, and you put it at a severe angle, it will appear as though it is being blown by a strong wind, or falling over. The feeling of tranquillity has changed to one of tension.

Curved lines give the feeling of a gradual flowing movement. A river is a great element that can move the eye gradually into a composition.

Spatial design (the arrangement of areas in a painting)

When working on paper or any two-dimensional plane spatial design is also very important. Try not to divide the paper equally in half; if working on a landscape, avoid making the sky one half and the land mass the other half. A more interesting design will be a proportion of three-quarters sky and one-quarter land, or a quarter sky and three-quarters land. Also avoid dividing it in half vertically. Keep taller objects towards the outer edges of the design and smaller ones towards the centre.

If producing a flower study, try an arrangement with the vase to one side of centre, with the taller flowers on the outer edge. The same design principle is often used by portrait painters, whether it is the head of a person or an animal. The head is frequently placed off centre, the face looking into a larger area than that behind the head.

Artists often use the technique of varying the spatial size of each area of a painting to create a more interesting composition.

Focus

Focus is another important aspect of design especially when creating a painting. If there are too many points of focus, the painting will be much weaker than if there is only a dominant one. Focus can be created by placement of a subject or by a light. Many artists use both.

A quick thumbnail exercise will illustrate the point. Start with a similar rectangle as before. Place a small dot anywhere in the rectangle. Immediately the focus is on that tiny dot. Now add several more dots of the

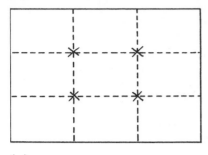

(a)

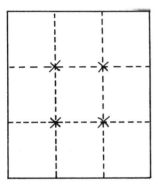

(b)

Figure 1.7

same size, placing them at irregular intervals within the rectangle. It is now impossible to focus on one in particular. Enlarge one of the dots and that point now becomes the focal point. Study paintings and photographs by well known artists and you will see how they use this device effectively. As I have said, light is often used to strengthen a focal point further. By making this point light and the surrounding area dark, more emphasis is in this area. A full moon in a star-filled sky is an excellent example of this.

Placement of the focal point has also to be considered. If it is placed too close to the edge of a painting, the composition will appear out of balance. A simple rule of thumb is to divide any format that you are considering for a painting into thirds (Figure 1.7). As an example, draw a small rectangle. Divide it into thirds both ways. The main subject can be placed at one of the four points of intersection, lending interest to the composition.

The following exercise will help you understand the basis of this principle. Draw out two small rectangles. Make a shape to represent a small cottage; it can be very simple. Position it at one of the lower recommended positions. Now repeat the process, placing the cottage at one of the higher points. You will find that the cottage will appear more dominant at this point. Angular or curved lines, such as paths, fences lines or grasses, can be used to draw the viewer's eye towards the subject. The mood of the design can be altered dramatically by changing the flow of these elements from straight to curved lines.

Colour design

I teach those without previous knowledge of painting to use just three colours: the three primaries, red, blue and yellow. It must be noted that there are, of course, several different reds, blues and yellows. It would take pages to explain and show their differences. A basic knowledge of colour theory is all that

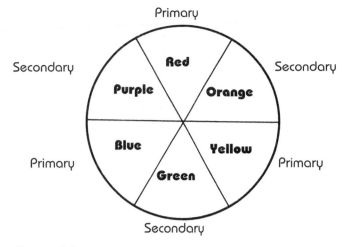

Figure 1.8

is required for the projects in this book, so I will keep this section as simple as possible.

Figure 1.8 shows the basis of colour, three primary and three complementary colours. Mixing all three primaries together in equal proportions will give a grey. Try this for yourself by mixing a grey in this way. If the grey turns a grey green add its complementary colour, red. If it tends to be more yellow add more blue and red (violet being its complementary colour). If it becomes more orange add a little blue. This will give you a good understanding of colour mixing.

While doing this exercise you may have mixed many colours. It will become apparent that a painting can be produced with many moods and colour variations, simply with these three colours. When using opaque colours such as acrylics, it will be necessary to include white in the colour palette. When using watercolours, I do not use white paint, but rely on transparent washes to create light tones. Many artists do use a watercolour white with very good results. When added to watercolours, it makes the colours more opaque, similar to gouache pigments.

I do not include a black in my palette either, but instead use colours like burnt umber or burnt sienna with vermilion or cadmium red and cobalt blue;

these, I feel, give far more interesting dark areas. It is important not to be tempted to put many colours together in one composition until one has more experience with colour combinations. By keeping to a minimal selection of colours the painting will always be harmonious.

The use of complementary colours is another important consideration when planning a painting. They can be used to draw attention to a specific area and to enliven a dull painting. Complementary colours used next to one another become vivid and appear to shimmer. Large areas with equal amounts of complementary colours next to one another will tend to vibrate too much. In a design of this nature, it is far better to have less of one complementary colour than the other. Having now briefly explained a few principles on design, it is up to one's personal taste whether or not to follow such principles. I find it exciting to watch people explore their own creative paths, but when teaching I would always recommend that a student starts with these basic rules. All of the foregoing can be used as exercises when teaching others.

Brush techniques

As several of the projects throughout the book require the use of an artist's brush, the following will help you brush up on your brushwork!

Some do's and don'ts

Do wash brushes after use. Water-based pigments have been suggested throughout this chapter, so clean up simply with water. When leaving brushes for any period of time after use, wash and dry them and lie them flat. Do not stand them handle first in a container while wet, or even damp. The water will seep back into the wooden handle and damage it.

Do not leave brushes standing in water for long. It will damage the bristles and, in time, loosen the ferrule (the metal bit).

After a period of time paint can settle in the base of the bristles and become quite hard. This can be removed by vigorously rubbing the base on a bar of soap and rinsing the bristles in warm water. This may have to be repeated more than once. A special soap is also available from an art materials supplier.

To obtain fine detail or filling in corners when glass painting, hold the brush in a vertical position when applying pigment. As long as it is of good quality, the largest brush will give fine detail.

If fine grasses or branches are required, use the brush almost vertically and lift the brush off the painting surface before finishing the stroke (the quicker the brush stroke, the better).

One-stroke brushes can also give fine detail by using the corner of the brush.

Larger surface areas can be covered with a round brush by applying paint with the brush laid on its side.

Scumbling is a method of applying paint to give a rough texture. It can be used as a background or as a glaze over a dried colour. A minimal amount of paint is used with the brush quite dry. The brush can be dried on a scrap piece of paper if it is loaded too much. It is used on its side with little pressure. (This is technique is useful for bricks, stonework, trees, etc.)

Texture can also be added to a surface by using an old toothbrush dipped in paint. Hold the brush horizontally, pointing at the work with the bristles up. The thumb is dragged across the bristles, spraying paint onto the work but not you, hopefully! It can get a little messy until you master the technique, but it is well worth the effort. A small natural sponge can also give an interesting texture. Use it with minimal colour and with a light application.

A straight line can easily be made with a brush. Place a ruler where the line is required. Tilt the ruler towards you at an angle of about 45 to 60 degrees, keeping the back edge on the work surface The angle of the ruler may have to be adjusted, depending on the size of the brush, to allow just the ferrule to slide along the ruler. Load the brush and run the ferrule along the lifted edge of the ruler. Keep the ruler tilted and the brush at a constant angle and pressure on the work surface. The ferrule should maintain contact with the ruler while the line is being formed.

When working in acrylics, the paint can be applied with a hard flat or round bristle brush or a palette knife. Both can give excellent impasto effects (thick layers of paint). This is well worth trying, as it frees up the work of people who may be painting in a restricted manner.

If a shaky hand is a problem, one hand can be steadied by holding it with the other. Another alternative is to make a support stick. This can be made from a broom handle cut to about 380 mm (15 in). Wrap strips of material at one end, cut a square or circular piece and wrap this over the material to make a pad; secure with string. This will prevent the stick from moving when leant on.

Painting

The foregoing deals with the watercolour painting as I have found it to be a lovely medium for older people to use. It is easy to clean spillages and there is no smell. Acrylics is another medium I recommend and is dealt with in chapter 2. There is a preconception that watercolour painting is very difficult and that alterations cannot be made. In this section, I will try to dispel such myths and explain some basic principles that will help when painting or instructing others using this medium.

Although watercolour paint is referred to as a transparent medium, some colours are less transparent than others. This does have an effect in mixing and when using the glazing technique.

Glossary of painting terms

- Hue – the identification of a colour, red, blue, etc.
- Tone or value – the degree of lightness or darkness

of a colour, tones or values are better seen in a black and white photograph.

- Chroma or intensity – this is the brightness of a colour.
- Wash – a layer of colour applied to a painting surface.
- Primary colours – red, yellow and blue are the primary colours, they cannot be made by mixing, and are the foundation from which other colours are mixed.
- Secondary colours – the resulting colour when two primary colours are mixed together.
- Complementary colours – the colour that is directly opposite another colour on the colour circle (see Figure 1.8).
- Glaze – a thin layer of paint applied over another.
- Wet-in-wet – pigment added to a layer of paint that is still wet.
- Negative shape – the area around a form.
- Aerial perspective – the impression of distance. This can be well observed in a landscape, the furthest distance seems relatively light with diminished colour; objects closer appear darker and brighter in colour.

Watercolour paper

As previously mentioned, watercolour paper is available in different weights (thickness) and in a variety of sizes in sheet form or pads. I have suggested that you use 300 gsm (140 lb), as this is readily available. The thinner weights do not stand up as well to 'lifting off' or a lot of 'scrubbing'. Both these techniques will be explained later. It is important to use watercolour paper for painting in this medium, as ordinary paper will not give the delicate washes and nuances of colour you can get with the correct paper. Student grade paper and pigment are available and quite acceptable, if your budget is limited. Most art stores carry a good selection of paper, pigment and brushes.

If you have purchased watercolour paper in sheet form you will need to cut it to fit the support; a quarter of a sheet is a convenient size. Before you cut the paper, you should first determine the correct side to paint on. The more expensive papers will have a watermark in one or more corner; hold the sheet up to the light and the side with the watermark readable the right way is the correct side. Both sides can actually be used but they do vary a little. When you have cut the paper, mark the right side of each cut sheet with a pencil mark. This will remind you later which is the correct side. If you are purchasing less expensive paper, it may not have a watermark. Ask the shop clerk at the time of purchase. The uppermost side of paper in pad form is quite obvious.

Stretching watercolour paper

Although some artists do not pre-stretch the paper, I recommend that it be done, especially when using lighter papers. If wet-in-wet painting is attempted on unstretched light paper it will buckle, giving annoying valleys for the paint to settle into.

The support needs to be about 50 mm (2 in) wider on all four sides than the watercolour paper.

Cut up strips of the gummed paper to fit the four sides of the watercolour paper, allowing a little extra so that the gummed paper is longer than each side. Put some water into a saucer, and have some scrunched-up paper towel or a small sponge to hand. Turn the watercolour paper over to the side that is not going to be painted on, and moisten this whole surface with the sponge or towel. Be careful not to saturate the paper. Let the paper absorb the water for a minute or so; do not leave it too long or the paper will dry out. Place the paper, damp side down on the board. As it is important to moisten the gummed paper evenly, I have found the following procedure works very well. Put the paper towel or sponge in the saucer of water, moisten the gummed paper by pulling a piece, gummed surface down, over the moistened material. A slight pressure on the back of the gummed tape will ensure that it picks up adequate water evenly.

Place the strips, as you moisten them, along each side of the watercolour paper – half of the width of the tape on the board and the other on the paper. Another piece of scrunched-up paper towel can be used to press the strips down securely. When all four strips are in place, allow the watercolour paper to dry completely. Check with the back of the hand: if the paper feels cool it is still wet.

Some watercolour painting do's and don'ts

- Do not apply colours directly from the tube or cake, mix colours in the palette first.
- Adding water to a pigment changes its tone or value, lightening it (changes the amount of lightness or darkness).
- To change the intensity of a colour (brightness), mix it with its complementary colour. (Red's complementary colour is green, blue's is orange, yellow's is purple. They are the colours directly opposite one another on the colour circle.)
- If a hard edge is wanted to an area, apply paint with the paper dry.
- If a soft edge is wanted apply paint with the paper damp.
- Dry each wash before applying another, unless you want the colours to mix on the paper.
- A hairdryer will speed up the drying process.

Further techniques

Do not mix more than three colours together or the final colour will be dull and 'muddy'; some artists actually use this colour mixing to great effect.

Start the painting with the lightest colours where possible. Add darker and more intense colours later. Keep the initial washes thin, with a high water-to-pigment ratio. Build the colours up with glazes, it is very important that each layer of colour be completely dry before applying another glaze. Watercolour paint is transparent, some colours more than others, so each layer that is applied affects the next. If too many dark layers or colours that are less transparent are applied the painting will become dull and lifeless. If this happens, the painting can be actually lightened by a lifting off method, described later.

Colours can be mixed on the paper, 'wet-in-wet', by adding more intense colours than those already painted (higher pigment to-water ratio) It is very important not to let the first layer of paint dry before adding more colour. If it is semi-dry, the colours will not mix. A delightful effect can be obtained by adding water to an already applied wet colour. They are sometimes referred to as 'back-runs'. Another effect that gives an interesting background to, say, a flower painting, is to sprinkle salt onto wet paint. Do not use a brush at this stage, just allow the painting to dry naturally. When the painting is dry the salt should be carefully removed, by shaking the paper or brushing with a household brush. The resulting starburst effect can be very interesting indeed. Keep salt away from your watercolour brushes and pigments.

To remove or diminish unwanted painted areas, first dry the painting thoroughly. Keep handy a clean piece of paper towel. With clean water moisten a brush and tap off the excess water. Rub the unwanted area with the damp brush; if it is a large area a sponge should be used. The applied paint should start to soften. While the area is still wet put the brush or sponge aside, lay the piece of paper towel on the wet area and with the heel or back of your hand, wipe it firmly in one direction over the paper towel. Lift the paper towel off and check if enough pigment has been removed. Repeat if more colour needs to be removed. Some colours stain more than others, so the process may have to be repeated several times. For very stubborn colours a small scrub brush or toothbrush could be used instead of the painting brush. Be aware that less expensive or thin watercolour papers will not stand up to this type of correction.

An exercise you would do well to try is to create a graduated wash, as this will be used in the landscape painting project in chapter 2. When trying to create the illusion of distance in a sky, it should be remembered that warmer and darker colours bring an area closer to the viewer. Likewise, cooler and lighter tones of colour will appear to be further away. So graduating a wash from warm and dark to cool and light-toned, will give one the feeling of distance in the sky. This is actually referred to as aerial perspective.

If you do not have any experience with the watercolour medium, I recommend that the following exercise be tried. Often, before artists start a painting, they will tone the painting support, i.e. the paper or canvas. This helps to suppress the fear of the blank surface, but more importantly, unifies the painting.

Watercolour painting exercise

1. Toning paper with a wash

Materials required:

- Pre-stretched watercolour paper
- One stroke watercolour brush 25 mm (1 in) or large round
- Watercolour pigment: vermilion
- Palette or saucers
- Water pot
- Paper towel
- Blocks or bricks

Stretch the watercolour paper and allow to dry thoroughly. The support board should be tilted up to allow the wash to bead up. In the palette mix a light vermilion wash by using plenty of water. When working with watercolours in large areas, always mix more paint than you think you will require. Running out of paint halfway through an application like this is definitely not what you want!

Load the brush with colour. Start the brush stroke off the paper at the top left (top right of the paper if you are left-handed), apply the pigment with a single horizontal stroke. Do not apply too much pressure or alter the pressure as you move the brush. Avoid lifting the brush or going back over the wash. As long as a good amount of watercolour is loaded in the brush and the support board is tilted enough, the line of colour will start to bead up at the lower edge. As soon as you have finished the stroke pick up more pigment in the brush and apply another stroke below the first. Overlap only the bottom edge of the first layer; the brush should just touch the bead as it moves across the paper. The two bands of watercolour will join together without leaving an overlap line. Continue applying paint in this manner until the bottom of the paper has been reached. Dry any excess paint that might occur at the right and left and bottom of the watercolour paper.

The following exercise will help you when painting in the traditional manner of foreground, middle ground and distance. Aerial perspective has to be really understood and applied.

2. Grading a wash

Materials required:

As in the previous exercise, but use cobalt blue instead of vermilion. Mix in the palette or saucer a fairly strong wash of cobalt blue, and lots of it.

With the paper stretched and dried, load the brush. Starting your brush stroke off the paper as described in the previous exercise.

Repeat the process with one more brush stroke. Before applying another brush stroke, add a little water to the wash. Stir the paint well and load the brush. As you brush this wash across, picking up the bead as before, you should notice that the colour is a little lighter. Do not worry if there is not a significant change, just carry on and finish the stroke. Add more water to the wash colour, and continue with another brush stroke. Repeat the diluting and brushing process until the bottom of the paper has been reached. Dry up any wet spots around the paper. The finished painting should gradually lighten towards the bottom of the paper.

This will give you a basis on which to start the watercolour project of the mountain scene in chapter 2.

Chapter 2

Drawing and painting

Drawing
Painting with watercolours
Painting with acrylics

Drawing

The section at the end of the book on patterns and designs includes line drawings that can be photocopied or traced, and transferred to another surface. However, the following projects will enable you to work from other images you may have available, whether they are photographs or outline drawings. The projects can be attempted by those in your care with good tactile skills, but help may be required when measuring and making the grids. People may just like to watch while you prepare the images.

Tip
Keep pencils sharp, the softer lead will need sharpening often so have a pencil sharpener at hand.

Project 1

Transforming a photograph to a line drawing

To make a line drawing of a photograph and to transfer it (same size) onto an A4 sheet of paper.

Materials required:
- One sheet of paper, A4 size
- Ruler
- 2H and 4B pencils
- Red pencil crayon
- One sheet of tracing paper
- One sheet of carbon paper
- A good photograph with high contrast

Procedure

The traced image can be used as your master copy, or it can be photocopied. Tracing paper is rather fragile and will tend to go brittle with age.

If you have not had any art training in perspective drawing, try this project with a photograph of a street scene. The lines you create will give you a basic understanding of the principles of perspective.

Make sure that the image, or the part of the image you select, will fit comfortably on an A4 sheet of paper. As you just want to end up with an outline drawing, you can use tracing paper to advantage here. Work on a flat firm surface and attach only the top or side of the tracing paper to the photograph or part that you are interested in. This will act as a hinge and allow you to lift up the tracing paper to check for detail when necessary. Using the red pencil crayon, carefully trace the image you require, checking that you have the relevant parts of the photograph traced before detaching the tracing paper.

While at this stage, you should try to simplify the detail, remembering that the completed drawing is to be used by the elderly, whose eyesight and hand coordination may not be at their best.

Place the traced image at the required position on the A4 sheet. Again, attach only the top or side of the tracing paper to the A4 sheet, placing the carbon paper between the tracing paper and sheet. Make sure you put the carbon paper transfer side down, or you will transfer your image to the back of the tracing paper. And yes, it has been done! With the 2H pencil, go over the red lines. You want to try to get a nice clean line transferred, so try not to go over the same line twice or you will get a thicker or even a double line. The red line will disappear and become a grey pencil line instead. Do not lean on the tracing paper with your hands or you will get some smudging transferred as well. Lift up the tracing paper from time to time and check that your line has transferred well. Before detaching the tracing paper, check once more that all of the image you require has been transferred.

Now that you have a line drawing of the original photograph, you may wish to make it more durable or darker for photocopying by going over the transferred image with a fine black felt-tipped pen. It can now be enlarged on a photocopier or 'squared up' as the following project will show.

You can use this method to assemble different images from a variety of sources, making interesting collages. The following 'squaring up' method of enlarging or reducing an image is a good exercise to go through with the older person, who can help or just watch the process. I have used it many times. This method of transferring images has been used for hundreds of years by mural and scenery painters. You may like to use it for something similar, or just to change the size of an original image.

Project 2
Changing the size of an image

To make a line drawing of a photograph and to transfer it in larger or smaller scale onto an A4 sheet of paper.

Materials required:
- One sheet of paper, A4 size
- Ruler
- 2H pencil
- One sheet of tracing paper, A4 size
- Photograph or line image

Procedure

You may wish to make the image smaller or larger, so the following will take you through a simple procedure to transfer the image to any size you choose; it could even be a wall! Find the centre of a side of the A4 sheet of tracing paper and make a pencil mark; do the same for the other three sides. From these centre points, mark each 15-mm interval out to the right and left edges. When you have completed all four sides, draw a straight line between corresponding points on opposite sides of the paper, using a 2H pencil. If you

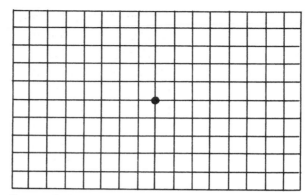

Figure 2.1

want to reuse the grid, use a waterproof fine line pen. You now have a grid of squares. Letter down one side and number across the other, just like you would find on a street or road map. It is a good idea to make the centre point larger so that you can find it easily (see Figure 2.1).

Trace an image from the pattern section of the book and secure it with masking tape to a flat surface. Position the centre of the grid approximately in the centre of the image and secure the grid at one edge only, so that you can lift it up from time to time to check details.

Using the 2B pencil draw the image onto the tracing paper. Keep the point of the pencil sharp, as it dulls quite quickly when used on tracing paper. You will notice that the lines you draw intersect the grid lines at various points. Setting this aside for the moment, secure the A4 sheet of paper on a flat surface, making sure that the image you are transferring fits proportionally on your paper (in other words if the image is wider than it is high, place the paper accordingly when you secure it to the working surface). Find the centre of all four edges and connect opposite points as before. You now have to decide what size you want the final image to be. Mark the longest side and place these points equally on either side of the centre line. Round them off to an even number. From your traced image note how many squares the longest side has and divide the new size into that same number of squares. Check the traced image once more and find the number of squares required for the other direction. Complete the new grid by measuring off from the centre line the same number of squares.

Your two grids should correspond by having the same number of squares in the area that you want to transfer. Number and letter the lines in the same way that you did on the master grid.

With your two grids alongside one another it is now just a matter of comparing where points intersect on the tracing paper grid and transferring them to your new grid. As you work through transferring the image you may want to join up these points as you go. On completion, you will have a line drawing that is a larger or smaller replica of the original image.

As in the previous project you can now transfer the newly sized image to any surface, or you can trace it to create another master without grid lines. This can then be photocopied if you wish.

If you want to reuse the master grid for another image, the first pencilled image can now be erased.

Tonal work and value study

When teaching drawing techniques I usually start with a project that involves tonal work or value studies, as it gives a good grounding to anyone wishing to draw in a realistic style. I find also that once this is understood, those starting to paint for the first time really appreciate the time spent in this area, as they begin to get good results quite quickly.

Project 3
Creating distance

To create a tonal drawing to show how different tones can give the illusion of distance.

Materials required:
- One sheet of paper A4 size
- Ruler 2H, 2B, 4B pencils

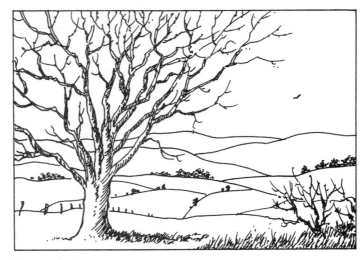

figure 2.2

Procedure

With reference to Figure 2.2 make a similar line drawing using your 2H pencil; use light pressure only. Starting with the sky, vary the tone from left to right, so that the sky is lightest on the left. Still using the 2H pencil, shade in the farthest mountain. Try to blend in this tone so that there is no outline of the mountain showing. Now do the same with the next farthest, but press a little harder so that the tone is a little darker. For the next hill use the 2B pencil and shade this a little darker than the last mountain, but don't make it too dark. The fields can be shaded with the 2H pencil at the farthest point, and with the 2B closer to you. You will now see that the lighter tones appear to recede and the darker ones appear to be closer. This is called aerial perspective, and is one of the fundamentals of landscape painting.

To complete the illusion, shade the tree with the 4B pencil. You will also notice that we have created a light source from the left, so the tree can be shaded lighter on the left and darker on the right. Add the cast shadow of the tree with the 4B pencil. The tree is drawn bigger than space allows, so it extends beyond the top of the sheet. You may notice that this adds to the feeling of space and pushes the distant mountains further away.

The last project introduced you to using different grades of pencil to produce varied tones. Next, we will use the same pencil grades to create form and more realism.

Project 4
Shading techniques

To create form using line shading.

Materials required:
- A4 size paper. Smooth drawing paper will give better results than a bond duplicating paper.
- 2H, 2B, 4B pencils

Procedure

Draw a leaf shape as shown in Figure 2.3 using a 2H pencil; use light pressure. Now shade in the whole shape using a curve to your line as shown. The lines should be close together. Try to maintain the same pressure as you do this so that you end up with a flat tone. The outline should now have disappeared. With the 2B pencil, cross-hatch some of your initial lines to give darker tones, again curving your stroke. Finally, holes and blemishes can be indicated using the 4B pencil (Figure 2.3b).

When doing tonal drawings a higher degree of realism can be achieved with more shading. If the entire form is covered with the correct tonal value it will replicate a black and white photographs.

Try this technique with other subjects that are easily available; you will be surprised how realistic they become. Remember give hard surfaces a sharp edge to the reflected light, while soft surfaces should have a gradual softening.

When finishing studies like this, it will be noticeable that the object will tend to 'float'. This can be remedied by placing a cast shadow at the base of the object. The shadow should be drawn with horizontal lines to indicate that it is placed on a flat surface.

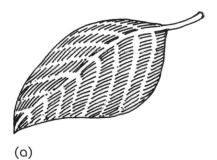

(a)

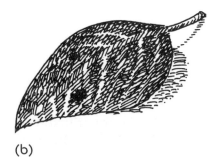

(b)

Figure 2.3

Project 5
To create form using dots (pointillism)

Materials required:
- Paper, A4 size – a smooth drawing paper will give better results than bond duplicating paper.
- 2H pencil
- Black fine line writing pen

In this exercise a form is going to be built up using a series of dots. You might like to try obtaining gradual tones from light to dark over a distance of about 75 mm (3 in), before you start the exercise. Using the pen in an upright position to obtain a small dot, be careful not to make a dash. Start placing dots a little distant from one another. As you move either left or right start to place the dots closer together. Continue the process of adding more dots as you move further away from your starting point. Place them closer and closer together until the dots begin to join. You may have to go back over the area to make the transition more gradual.

When working with people with poor eyesight the dots could be larger. You will have to hold the finished artwork further away to see the effect.

Now apply this technique to shape the apple; see how the form is created by the varying distance of the dots to one another. The more gradual the spacing of the dots, the more realistic the completed form will appear (Figure 2.4).

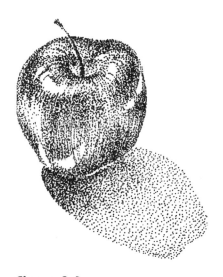

Figure 2.4

Project 6
Negative shapes

To create a form using negative shapes. You might find this terminology a little strange but it is often used by artists where light shades and colours are silhouetted against a dark background. It is often used to strengthen a design and give prominence to a particular area.

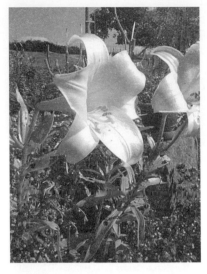

(a)

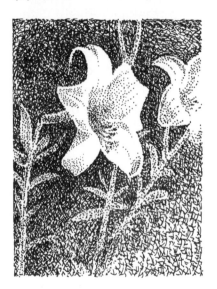

(b)

Figure 2.5

Materials required:
- Paper, A4 size – smooth drawing paper will give better results than bond duplicating paper.
- 2H, 2B pencils
- Black fine line writing pen
- Felt-tipped pens (optional)

Procedure

From the lily drawing in the section at the end of the book on patterns and designs, trace or copy it onto the working sheet. Refer to the photograph of the lily (Figure 2.5a), noting the delicate changes of tone. Using the pen, start adding dots as in the previous project. Work again from the lightest to the darkest tones; remember, it is best to stay on the light side to begin with. You can always add more dots if you feel an area needs to be darker, or if the transition is not gradual enough.

Once you have finished the lily form, use more dots to form the stems and leaves; note these shades are much darker than the lily petals. Referring to Figure 2.5b you will notice that an interesting background has been created by using an overlapping X stroke. The background is not the complicated background as in the photograph, but simply a variety of tones, darker than the blossom and leaves. As more contrast was wanted around the main lily head the background was made much darker here than at the extremities of the design. This was simply done by criss-crossing more X's on top of one another. The area with more contrast automatically creates a focus. Using a variety of coloured felt-tipped pens when working on a background like this creates a startling contrast to the white lily.

Painting with watercolours

The following projects will enable you to understand better the principles of watercolour painting. From these exercises it is hoped that you will create your own designs and help those around you to develop theirs. The projects deal with a traditional approach – putting in a foreground, middle ground and background. Also included is glazing, or veil painting as it is called by art therapists. When working 'wet-in-wet' or painting in large areas, it is advisable to stretch the paper. The procedure for this and how to produce flat and graded washes can be found in chapter 1.

Project 7
Watercolour painting using one colour (mono-chromatic)

Materials required:
- Board with stretched watercolour paper
- Bricks or blocks, two required
- One stroke brush, 25 mm (1 in)
- Watercolour pigment, cobalt blue
- Glass jar
- Water pot

Procedure

This process involves painting graded washes to form a series of hills and valleys. In the glass jar mix a small amount of pigment with a lot of water to give a very pale blue. Set the painting board on the bricks to give a tilt.

Charge the brush with coloured water and start the brush stroke off the paper. Keep the brush moving horizontally and do not lift it off the paper until it is clear of the tape at the other side of the sheet. A bead should have appeared along the bottom of the brush stroke. Recharge the brush and repeat the process, aiming to just pick up the bottom of the bead with the next brush stroke. Remember, overlapping it will result in a line being produced, and not touching it will create a white space.

Charge the brush with clean water and repeat the brush stroke as described. Continue this procedure

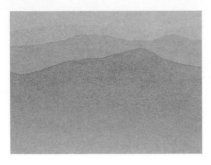

Figure 2.6

until the bottom of the page has been reached, picking up the bead each time. Be prepared to tilt the board a little more if a bead does not form, but not too much or the liquid colour might run down, leaving a vertical streak on your painting. Now dry the paper thoroughly.

Add a very small amount of pigment to the pale blue, just enough to darken it slightly. Charge the brush and start another brush stroke off the paper. The second wash needs to begin a little way down from the top of the painting, where the colour of the first wash starts to lighten.

This time, still taking the brush across the dry page in a horizontal direction, as you paint, move the brush up and down to create mountain forms, which will be silhouetted against the previous lighter wash. Recharge the brush and pick up the bead again as you move across the paper. Recharge the brush, with clean water this time, and repeat the painting process. You can level out the brush stroke now; continue the clear water wash until the bottom of the painting has been reached. Dry thoroughly.

The paint needs to be darkened slightly for each new wash (see Figure 2.6) by adding more pigment. Repeat the painting and drying process. If you have enough space on your page to paint four or five mountain ranges, so much the better. Each successive mountain range should give the appearance of gradually coming towards you out of the distance.

To create a painting with a more dramatic mood to it, use vermilion or a light red as the initial wash (background) colour. This will set the mountains against a blazing red sky.

Project 8

To create a watercolour painting of the landscape scene in Figure 2.2

Materials required:
- 2B pencil
- Watercolour paper A4 size (pre-stretched)

- Watercolour pigments – cobalt blue, cadmium yellow medium, vermilion
- Watercolour brushes – No 8, No 3 (a single stroke brush is optional)

Tips

1. Stirring the watercolour paint from time to time will help prevent the colours from separating.
2. Cadmium yellow is not as transparent, use it as thinly as possible.
3. When drying the paper with a hairdryer hold the dryer at an angle to the paper, and do not overdry, especially around the taped edges. Overdrying can cause the tape to crack off, necessitating a re-stretching of the paper.
4. Test for dryness by touching the paper gently with the *backs* of the fingers (not the front, where the oils in the skin are concentrated). A dry paper should have a smooth, flat surface. Make sure that the watercolour paper is thoroughly dry before commencing. It will probably help if the composition is drawn. Use the 2B pencil for this, and do not press hard as you do not want a dark indented line.

The support board should be tilted to allow the wash to bead up. A light blue-grey wash should now be mixed, using cobalt blue and a small amount of vermilion. Make sure there is enough colour mixed to cover the entire sheet. The No 8 or single stroke brush can now be loaded with paint. Starting at the top left of the paper, or top right if you are left-handed, take the brush lightly across the paper in a single smooth horizontal stroke. Follow the instructions in chapter 1 on creating a graduated wash. It is important that the quality of the wash in the lower portion of the sky is a very light tone, and the colour is of low intensity.

A slightly darker tone can now be made by adding a little more cobalt blue and vermilion to the mixture that is left. More water may also have to be added. The colour should be predominantly blue, and the tone just a little darker than the sky.

Once the paper has dried thoroughly, the distant mountain can be laid over the sky using the No 3 brush. As the overlap method of painting is to be used, the lower edge of this form should be softened with clean water. This will prevent a hard edge appearing when the next layer is painted over it.

The brush should be cleaned in water; the excess water is removed by tapping the ferrule of the brush on the side of the water pot. The bottom edge of the mountain can now be softened by running the moist brush along it. If too much water is used it will tend to run up into the previous wash and cause a 'back run'. This will dry as a light stain with a hard edge, something that needs to be avoided in this particular exercise.

Before another layer of paint is added, the painting should be totally dry.

More cobalt blue and vermilion should be added to the water, making it a little darker and more intense. This will be the colour for the second mountain range. It can now be laid in, following the pencil lines, overlapping the distant mountains, and painted down to the horizontal line of the mid-ground fields. Softening the lower and right-hand edges will allow the third form to be painted over the top, without the overlap showing.

When the painting is again completely dry, the third and final mountain can be added. As this can be considerably closer than the second range, a change of colour is in order. Cadmium yellow can be added to the paint as well a little more cobalt blue. This will change the colour to a blue green. It should not be too bright as the form still should look as though it is in the distance. The colour may have to be modified with some vermilion, to reduce the intensity. When laid over the second wash, three ranges should be distinguishable, receding into the distance.

The colour for the fields can now be mixed. By adding more yellow and blue, the colour will move towards stronger green. By keeping the distant pasture cooler (more blue) than the foreground, the space or depth in the painting will increase. The colours can be modified in the palette and tried on a scrap of paper until they look right.

As well as the foreground being a warmer green, a few details like spikes of grass or a bush can strengthen the foreground. This sort of detail should not be included in the mid-ground area, as the feeling of distance will be lost.

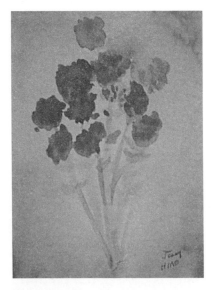

Figure 2.7

Project 9

To create a wet-in-wet painting using the flower design in Figure 2.7

Materials required are as used in project 7.

Make sure that the stretched paper is thoroughly dry before commencing.

Draw the flower forms lightly. Wet-in-wet paintings tend to lead the painter in unplanned directions, with the possibility of interesting 'accidents' happening along the way. So a detailed drawing is not required.

In the palette or dish mix up a dilute wash of cadmium yellow. In another dish mix up cadmium yellow and a little vermilion. This wash should have more pigment to water than the first mixture. These washes will be used to create a background for the flowers.

The support should hold the painting surface flat or with the top edge very slightly raised. The first wash can now be applied to the background with a diagonal brush stroke using the number 8 brush. Ensure that the painter starts and finishes the brush stroke off the paper. Before this wash starts to dry, the other wash should be painted, again in the same diagonal direction. To give a variation to the background, it should be painted where the first wash finished, or between areas first painted.

The colour will blend with the first wash nicely if it is laid in when it is still wet.

While the painting is drying a little vermilion needs to be added to the second wash to make it more intense. While the background wash is still wet, a small amount of this stronger pigment can be touched into the flower shapes using the number three brush. There should be no need to paint the shapes of the flower, as the pigment should spread on contact. If it tends to spread too much, it means that the background or the brush is too wet. This application should not be modified at this point, but be left to dry a little more. This procedure should then be tried again. Be aware that if the painting is left to dry for too long, the pigment will not flow when applied.

In the palette more vermilion needs to be added to this wash and the colour will be get much brighter. Again, while the painting is still wet, this pigment should be applied to the centres of some of the flowers. By not adding this to all of the flowers, some of the forms will appear to be closer or at different angles from others, giving an interesting depth to the painting. The colour for the stems can be made by adding a little cobalt blue to the palette of the last wash. As the background will probably be almost dry the stems, when painted in, will be quite well defined. They could be taken right out of the bottom of the painting or left as shown in the photograph. Leaves can now be added, using different greens made up from all three colours. The stems and leaves could have a variation of tone and colour to give them added dimension and gesture.

Project 10
Painting trees and foliage

Materials required are as given in the preceding watercolour projects.

Support the sheet of pre-stretched and dried watercolour paper at an angle of approximately 30 degrees, and lightly draw in the shape of the tree (see Figure 2.8a) and then the background detail.

In the palette mix cobalt blue and a touch of vermilion. The tone should be quite pale, so add plenty of water. It is always easier to darken a painted area than to lighten it. The sky can now be painted, using the graduated wash technique. Remember a loaded brush is required when trying to achieve gradated wash effects. Always paint right across the paper without stopping. If you have the correct amount of coloured water in the brush, a bead will form at the lower edge as you apply the paint. Dilute the colour with a small amount of water to reduce the tone a little before applying the next brush stroke. Do not wait too long as the bead will start to dry. Recharge your brush and apply the wash in the same manner as before, just picking up the bead remaining from your last brush stroke. Do not overlap the bead

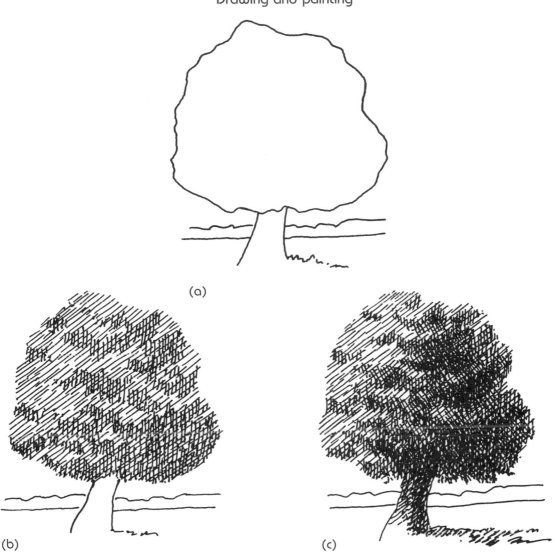

(a)

(b)   (c)

Figure 2.8

as this will result in stripes. Repeat the procedure for the next brush stroke, lightening the tone again by adding water. Continue painting in this manner down to the line of the fields in the distance. Paint right across the pencilled-in tree. If you need to make any alterations, they should be done at this stage. Dry the painting first before attempting any changes. If you feel that the sky is too dark, lighten it by using the lifting-off technique. If too light, apply another layer of washes. Dry the painting thoroughly each time before proceeding.

Add cadmium yellow to the wash to change it to a yellow-green. This can be laid in where the fields are shown. The foreground can be painted with more detail and colour. Paint right across the tree as you did with the sky. The distant trees can be added, with a light tone of blue to put them in the distance. A touch of vermilion will grey it a little if it is too intense. These distant forms should not have any detail.

At times you may want to lift colour in certain areas. This could well be the case here as the foliage on the left of the tree and tree trunk will need to be much lighter than the right side. If you feel that your painting is too dark in these locations, try the lifting-off technique described in chapter 1. Make sure that the painting totally dry and that you have a jar of clean water and paper towel handy. Moisten a round brush, tapping off any excess water. Paint the water over the tree and the trunk, and scrub at it if there is a lot of pigment. While still wet, lay the paper towel over the area and with the heel of your hand lightly but firmly smooth the paper down onto the painting. Lift it immediately; the area should now be much lighter. If it is not, dry the paper and repeat the process.

The foliage of the tree can now be painted using a yellow-green. All of the foliage should be covered. The diagonal lines in Figure 2.8b refer to this. This colour should be dried before adding more colour.

In the palette mix a darker green by adding more blue to the existing wash. The next darker green can now be laid over the first wash. As the light source is from the left of the tree, this area should not be painted further. The paint should be applied in the area as shown in Figure 2.8b by the vertical lines. A third colour needs to be mixed for the darkest green. As this will be in the shaded side of the tree, add a little more blue to the mixture. Refer to Figure 2.8c for the final effect.

The colour for the tree trunk can now be mixed. Start by mixing vermilion and cobalt blue with a good deal of water; this will make a light grey. This should now be applied to the entire trunk. In a small dish or part of the palette, mix cobalt blue and vermilion with just a little water. Apply this as soon as possible to the shadow side of the tree, mixing it wet-in-wet. If it does not appear to be dark enough, more cobalt blue can be added directly into left side of the tree trunk. At this time the shadow of the tree can be laid in, connecting the tree and shadow nicely.

Painting with acrylics

Painting with acrylics can be refreshingly simple. This medium has an opaque quality that can give the unskilled painter renewed confidence in his painting ability. It means that, unlike watercolours, acrylic pigment can be painted over to correct mistakes. It is a fairly recent medium to appear on the art scene, but its versatility and durability has earned it a permanent place as a painting medium. The paint will adhere to virtually any surface, with little preparation. It is water based so it mixes readily with water, and clean up is odour free. It has a painterly quality comparable to oil paint, and similar application techniques. This includes the use of soft and hard brushes such as synthetic and hog hair as well as application with a painting knife. I like the feel of painting in acrylics with hard bristle brushes and would suggest that you try them. They are well worth purchasing, as they are hard wearing and relatively inexpensive.

It is less tiring for older people to sit and paint at a table, than to stand or sit at an easel. The painting support can then be propped at a slight angle on the table, and work can be undertaken much like a watercolour project. When working in this position, long-handled brushes associated with hard bristle brushes are awkward to use, so I recommend that short-handled brushes be purchased, or the long ones cut down a little.

The painting surface can be wood, paper, card or a canvas board. A good variety of sizes, already primed, are available from your art supplier. The painting surface should always be primed before commencing a painting. This can be done with any acrylic-based primer.

I have used acrylic paint successfully with residents who have difficulty controlling watercolour paint. One of the drawbacks of the medium is that the pigment dries very quickly. However, a retarding agent can be mixed with the paint before application, slowing the drying rate substantially.

In chapter 1, I described how to modify watercolours to make colour less intense by adding the complementary colour, and also how to change the value of a colour by adding water to make it lighter. With acrylics, one adds white to change the value of the colour, thus making it lighter. The colour's brightness is modified by adding its complementary colour. If all this sounds too much to take in at one go, the projects that follow will clarify the points one by one. Acrylic paint has a similarity to watercolours in as much as it can be thinned with water and used as a transparent wash. But in my opinion it does not give the subtle nuances that watercolour is capable of. The medium is ideal for outdoor murals as it is water-resistant and does not peel or crack. There are also several additives that can increase the creative possibilities of acrylics. These include texture gels such as sand and pumice, as well as a modelling paste for heavy impasto work. The completed work can be varnished to give it a gloss, matt or satin finish.

If a retarding agent is not used, the following practice will help slow the drying rate of the paint on the plate. Place a piece of paper towel on the plate. Dampen the towel with a little water and lay out the colours directly on it. If the colours are left for just a short time they will start to form a skin, especially in a warm environment. Cover them with an upturned plate of the same size to help prevent this.

If there is paint left over from a painting session it

can be returned to the jar, or if tube paint has been used, a small container such as a 35-mm film cannister, makes an excellent storage pot. A dab of the paint on the outside of the lid will identify the contents nicely.

Project 11
Painting an English landscape

Materials required:
- Acrylic paint: vermilion, cobalt blue, cadmium yellow medium, burnt umber, titanium white
- Brushes, acrylic flat, sizes 2, 4, round No 4
- Palette or dinner plate
- Paper towel
- Water pot
- Support – primed canvas board or heavy card

Procedure

If you do not have the colours as recommended, others can be used. It is important that they are the three primary colours plus an earth colour.

If a drying retarder is not used, completely cover the palette with a piece of paper towel. Dampen it with water and put the acrylic pigment around the edge, directly on the moistened paper towel. Cover the pigment when not in use.

Use a clean brush or painting knife when taking colour for mixing, the original colours will then stay fresh and unmodified by the others. Always mix the colours in the centre of a palette or plate.

As a white painting surface can be somewhat overwhelming for a beginner, I suggest that a thin wash of colour be laid over the entire painting area. A suggested colour mix would be a very small amount of burnt umber with cadmium yellow and plenty of water. Brush this over the painting surface and leave to dry. Apart from diminishing the white, it will harmonize the entire painting,

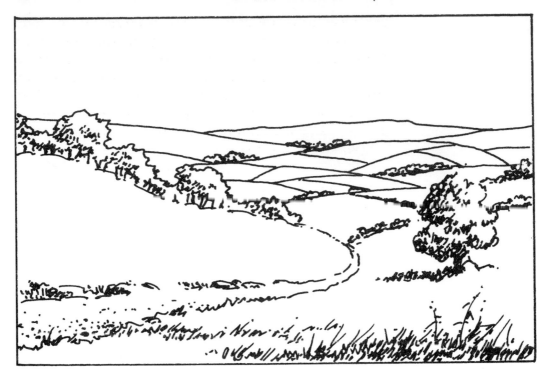

Figure 2.9

especially if it is allowed to show through a little when other colours are applied.

Refer to Figure.2.9, and lay out the landscape using cobalt blue well diluted, applied with the small round brush. When working on landscapes, I usually work from the top of the painting down, blocking in the shapes of the land masses. 'Blocking in' refers to the organization of shapes and is done with thin applications of paint. At this stage detail is not important, just concentrate on getting the shapes and values organized. It is important that the composition is balanced, value wise. If the painting is too dark at one side, it will feel lop-sided. Add a small dark area to the opposite side of the painting to counterbalance it. Squinting is a good way to see the values better. Remember values are just the amount of dark and light, they have nothing to do with colour. Once the painting has been blocked in and the paint is dry, you can start applying more pigment, concentrating on the colour. As you will not have a colour study to go by, colours will have to be guessed at. This is not as difficult as one would imagine. Keep the sky light by using cobalt blue mixed with a little white. It should be a little warmer and darker at the top of the painting, getting cooler and lighter as the sky recedes in the distance towards the horizon. To cool the blue, just add the tiniest amount of burnt umber; to lighten it add white. Do not add too much water now, just enough to keep the pigment fluid. Acrylics are quite opaque when mixed with a minimal amount of water, so mistakes and changes can be easily painted over. For the distant hills, mix a cool blue, it needs to be a little darker than the sky, or the hills will not be seen. It should not, however, be too dark or too bright or the hills will jump forward. To obtain a feeling of distance in a painting this rule of thumb should be considered: light, cool and dull colours seem to recede; dark, warm and bright colours come forward. This is the basis of aerial perspective in landscape painting. If the distant colour is not quite right, it can always be adjusted later. It is difficult to get the colour right first time, unless you are very experienced. Colours also appear to change when seen alongside other colours, so be prepared for some adjustment later.

The patchwork of fields can now be painted. Select different colours of greens and yellows. The furthest fields should not be too bright or contrast too much, or they will jump forward. Colours of the fields closer to the mid-ground should now be a little warmer; adding a little red will do this.

The field on the left can now be painted. Try to create some distance from the closer part to the furthest, by using the warm and cool technique just described. The group of trees at the top of the hill can now be added. Do not add too much detail, as this will have a similar effect as bright colours and bring them forward. Paint them as a mass without showing any individual leaves. A tree trunk or two could be shown if the painting is reasonably large.

The field to the right can now be completed. As the field reaches down to the bottom of the painting, this is a good opportunity to add some detail. Once the field is laid in with brighter greens and yellows in the foreground, add some grasses with the small brush. When this area is dry, add dots of pure yellow and red to represent wild flowers.

Next put in the road; again use the aerial perspective technique to create distance. The oak tree can now be tackled; the paint should be dry enough to draw the shape with a pencil if necessary. Create a light side to the right of the tree with yellow/green. A shadow can be painted at the base of the tree trunk which will direct the viewer's eye to the left, onto the road and then into the picture.

To determine if the painting is balanced, set it a little distance away from you and half close your eyes; you will see if any adjustment is necessary. If there appears to be more weight on one side of the painting than the other, then it is not balanced. Adjust the painting by lightening or darkening the area concerned.

Chapter 3

Working with paper

Collages
Mobiles
Paper beads
Decoupage
Paper flowers

The following projects can be used to make decorations for a room, given as gifts to young relatives or sent to a children's hospital ward. They would also make ideal fund-raising items.

Collages

When using a large format size for a paper collage, the support should be heavier than standard weight copier paper. This will help to prevent buckling. Once completed, the collage could be framed either with or without glass.

Different materials as well as paper can be used in a collage to give a very interesting three-dimensional effect. One could use pasta, beans, scraps of material, scrunched-up tissue paper, etc.; but please note when using this type of heavier material, a stronger support is required, such as hardboard or heavy card as used for packing boxes. Stronger PVA glue should also be used to ensure that the pieces do not fall off when the collage is held or mounted vertically.

Project 1
Flower collage

To create a flower design collage.

Materials required:
- Heavy paper or card, A4 size
- 2B pencil
- Several old magazines
- Wallpaper glue, diluted PVA glue or glue stick
- Scissors
- Large bowl, I use a dog food bowl
- Small paint brush

Procedure

Referring to Figure 3.1 roughly sketch out the outline of the collage onto the card.

Get the person or people you are working with to select coloured pages from magazines. Cut up the pages into random sizes of about 30 mm to 40 mm ($1\frac{1}{4}$ in to $1\frac{1}{2}$ in) across. Try to make them different

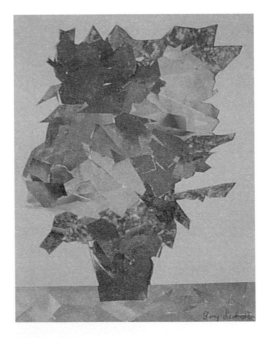

Figure 3.1

shapes. Sort them into their respective colours and put them into different trays; I find that paper plates work very well for this. As you will be cutting up photographs as well as blocks of colour, the pieces will not all be solid colours. But try to get them sorted into some order so that you can find different colours easily.

I let the person with whom I am working select the colours. Start with the background and suggest a variety of neutral colours or those that are not too bright. This will ensure that the chosen flower colours stay prominent in the composition. As the clippings are glued down, make sure that the pieces overlap so that none of the support paper shows. The background can be filled in, until all that is showing is the pencil lines of the flower shapes, vase and table. It is not important to be too accurate for when these forms are filled in with clippings, pieces should be placed so that they overlap the background slightly.

I drop the cuttings into the bowl to soak a little; they can easily be picked out with the brush and placed in position. If you find this gluing process too messy, a glue stick works well.

When the background is complete, the colours for the table and the vase need to be selected, and the clippings glued in place. When completed, the flower shapes can then be started.

In order to get some form into the flowers, consider where a light source might be coming from, perhaps from the top and a little to the left of the composition. Use the lighter shades of the chosen colour in this area, and darker shades of the colour towards the bottom and right of the flower shape. Experiment a little by just laying some cuttings down without gluing them. The pieces can be secured with the glue when an arrangement has been decided upon. The clippings should be overlapped when they are applied. It may be necessary to cut the clippings smaller if more realism is wanted, or if intricate shapes are required. Be careful not to cut them too small or you might create handling problems.

Different colours can be used for the various flowers. All the flower shapes need to be covered at this time.

Leaf shapes could be cut out from photographs that are predominantly green. Added to the flower arrangement, they give the overall design a more natural look. Flower colours can be added over some of the leaves so that the leaves appear to be below the flowers. Other leaves could overlap the flowers. A little direction and help may be required by you to tidy up the composition, but I have found that usually the completed collage is better left as the person working on it intended. The overall effect is one of a glorious impressionistic colour scheme. An example of another paper collage design is shown in Figure 3.2.

Many interesting collages can be produced using designs of animals, birds and landscapes. I have included a few possibilities in the section on patterns and designs. The design could be completed using as close to realistic colours as one can get from the selection of clippings that are available or, alternatively, it could have a totally imaginary colour scheme.

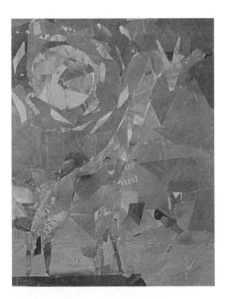

Figure 3.2

Collages do not have to be limited to paper, they can also include fabric such as netting, string, ribbon, lace and material scraps. One can also take this method of creating pictures a step further and produce assemblages. These are collages made from objects that are found such as seashells, small pebbles and dried leaves. Clock and watch parts make wonderful designs and are a great way to recycle unwanted articles. They are constructed in a similar fashion to collages but a much heavier support is required such as 10-mm ($\frac{3}{8}$-in) plywood. A strong PVA glue will also have to be used to attach the heavier pieces. Some parts may need to be nailed in position.

Mobiles

Patterns for mobiles can be found in the pattern section at the end of book.

Making mobiles is another way to stimulate the creative involvement of older people. Mobiles can be used to quickly add colour and interest to an otherwise dull and uninteresting room or space. When hung, the mobiles should rotate freely with the natural air circulation.

A mobile can be made from thin card or paper, depending on its size. Small items can be made from paper, but larger forms should be made from card, or they will tend to curl and not hang very well.

I recommend that you involve the participant at the start of the project, showing possible designs that could be used. If the person or people you are working with need a starting point, draw out a design on the card, either from the designs available or from one you've made yourself. Simple forms work well for mobiles, as they are usually viewed from a distance. They are also easier to colour.

When colouring the mobiles, bright colours found in packs of felt-tipped pens work very well; they are easiest to handle and apply. You could also try using watercolours or poster paints, but as they have a high water content, you will find that they curl the thinner paper and even the card if applied very wet. To give them a more decorative appearance, especially for the Christmas season, one can glue sequins, glitter, or small pieces of foil or silver paper onto the design. (I have used empty crisp packets, cut into small pieces, as they usually have a silver coating on the inside.) Make sure that they are attached securely by using white glue, diluted one part water to one part glue.

If felt-tipped pens are used for making a bird mobile, for example, one can suggest feathers by using line strokes in the direction of the bird's form. Review the different shading techniques in chapter 1.

Project 2
Bird mobile

To create a bird mobile.

Materials required:
- 2B pencil
- Three sheets of A4 white craft card
- One felt-tipped pen pack of assorted colours
- Scissors
- White cotton thread

Procedure

From the section on patterns and designs at the end of the book select the bird forms. They could be enlarged or reduced to make the mobile more interesting. If one is to construct several mobiles using this design, copy or transfer the designs onto pieces of thick card. These can then be cut out to make templates. It is then very easy to transfer these shapes onto the working white card by tracing around the edges with a pencil.

When the designs have been transferred, they can be cut out ready for colouring.

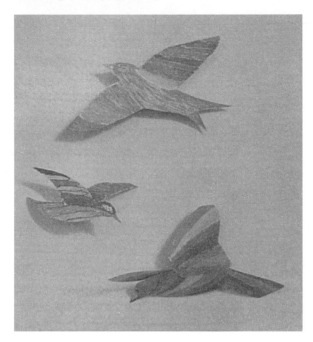

Figure 3.3

I suggest that a design be drawn onto the working cut-out so that the participant will have some colour and lines to follow (see Figure 3.3). There are usually many bird reference books at your local public library that will give you some design ideas. It is always a good idea to keep the design simple, making sure it suits the capabilities of the person you are working with. The birds can be made to look realistic, using true-to-life colours, or, again, the colours could be purely imaginative, with bright and unusual colour schemes. I prefer the latter as they will then certainly brighten the dullest corner of a room.

Once all the designs have been completed, remembering that both sides of each form need to be coloured, they can be attached to the mobile structure and hung up. Put the largest forms in the uppermost part of the mobile and the smaller ones in the lowest. Make sure that each form moves freely before securing the mobile in position.

To create an interesting three-dimensional look to this type of mobile follow the construction procedure set out in Figure 3.4.

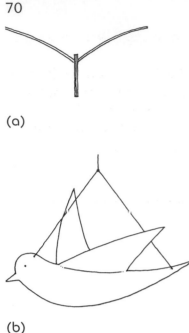

(a)

(b)

Figure 3.4

Cut out two of each of the bird shapes as in the preceding project. Set aside in pairs. As each pair is to be glued together at the body and not at the wings, mark the gluing area with an 'x.' Colour the forms as previously explained. Do not glue together until the forms are coloured. Naturally, the area to be glued does not require colour. Remember that each wing will have to be coloured on both sides. When the colouring has been completed, glue the body area together. As the wings are not glued together they can be bent downwards (see Figure 3.4a), creating a more realistic bird appearance. Attach cotton thread as indicated (Figure 3.4b) and join each bird shape together as previously instructed. Make sure that each bird form can rotate freely before hanging the completed mobile.

Another hanging configuration is to use fairly heavy wire to form lateral rods from which to suspend the forms. Cut a piece of wire 300 mm (12 in) long, turn both ends to form a hook and curve the wire slightly. This will be the first rod. Make two more rods from wire cut to 150 mm (6 in). Hook and curve the ends of these rods as you did the first. Lie the three rods on a table and set the bird forms in position without tying them to the rods. In this way you can see whether the forms will rotate freely without touching one another.

The bird mobile forms could also be used for a collage. Instead of colouring with felt-tipped pens, apply colourful pieces of paper, as in the preceding project on collages. Trim off the excess paper to give a clean contour.

Other forms that work very well as mobiles are stars, butterflies and leaves. Of course your imagination is the best resource; many ideas can be gleaned by thumbing through books and magazines.

Paper beads

Making paper beads is a craft activity that does not require any special skills. The finished product is attractive and hard wearing, making it a suitable gift for children or for an adult.

I would advise that the beads produced in this manner should not be given to very young children, as they might put them in their mouths.

I have suggested that standard felt-tipped colouring pens be used in the following project. Varnish is applied to make the beads waterproof and to give them a lustrous finish. If you do not want to varnish the beads, waterproof felt-tipped pens can be used.

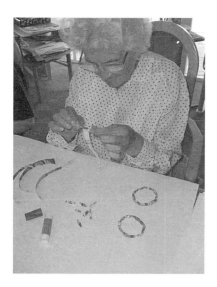

Project 3
Bead bracelet

Making a paper bead bracelet.

Materials required:
- Copy paper, A4 size (three or four sheets)
- 2B pencil
- A variety of coloured felt-tipped pens
- Glue stick
- Six bamboo skewers cut to about 130 mm (5 in)
- No 1 knitting needle
- White, 2 mm ($\frac{1}{16}$in) diameter round elastic
- Scissors
- Clear varnish
- Small brush for varnishing
- Old magazine
- Lid of egg box

Procedure

Draw a design on the paper; sweeping or zigzag lines are suitable (see Figure 3.5). Several sheets need to be prepared in this way, depending on the number of beads required. Using felt-tipped pens, get the participant(s) to colour the design using colours of his or her choice. Get them to try different colour schemes so that the result is one of multi-

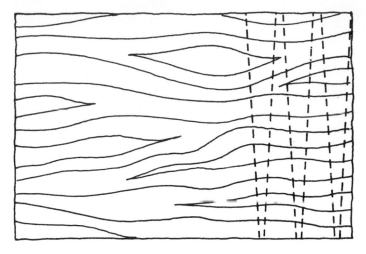

Figure 3.5

colours or perhaps a combination of two colours only. I find this part of the project interesting as the completed colouring alone can be a work of art.

Plain coloured sheets could also be used. You will find that colouring the sheets as previously described will give very colourful beads.

When all of the sheets have been coloured, they now need to be cut into tapered strips. It will depend on the participants' skills whether they are able to cut them up. Cut across the narrow width of the paper tapering the cut as shown by dotted lines in Figure 3.5. The more acute the angle, the more the design will show. When making beads for bracelets, the widest end should be no more than 15 mm ($\frac{5}{8}$in). For a small wrist, this size will lie evenly and attractively, 10 to 11 beads will make a bracelet to fit a child's wrist.

Store the cut pieces in a container, as they tend to curl and roll about. Each strip has now to be glued and rolled, so you will need the bamboo stick and glue-stick handy. Taking one of the pieces of cut strips, lay it, coloured side down, onto a page in the magazine. The paper strip will show up better when it is laid onto a dark or coloured background. Get the participant to glue the paper starting about 10 mm ($\frac{3}{8}$in) in from the widest end. (This will make it easier for the bead to be removed from the stick.)

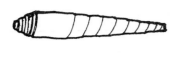

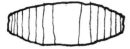

Figure 3.6

When the strip has been covered with glue, the widest end should be held against the stick with the coloured side out and towards the person. Start to roll it around the bamboo stick. You may find that someone with poor tactile ability may need help in getting it started, as it needs to be rolled quite tightly. Continue rolling until the strip is completely rolled and glued to itself. Check to see that the end has adhered to properly, re-glue if necessary. To ensure that the completed bead shape is reasonably symmetrical, keep the paper strip centred while rolling (see Figure 3.6). If the bead is lop-sided, hold the largest end of the bead between the thumb and first finger and push the narrow end against the nail of your other thumb. If this is done quickly, before the glue has completely dried, the rolled paper will move enough to make the bead shape more even. Roll all the paper strips into beads before going to the next stage.

For each bracelet, one bead has to be made with a larger centre. This is to hide the knot of the elastic that is tied after threading the beads. To make a larger hole, use a darning needle instead of a cocktail stick when wrapping a paper strip.

It is more convenient to varnish the beads before threading them onto the elastic. Put a few beads onto a cocktail stick leaving the ends of the stick protruding. This will allow the sticks to be supported over the eggbox lid as shown (see Figure 3.7). Apply a coat of varnish and leave to dry; apply four more

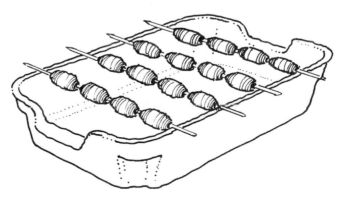

Figure 3.7

layers of varnish, letting each coat dry thoroughly before applying the next. The varnish may cause the beads to bind to the stick. If this happens, gently rotate the bead until it becomes free.

All that is now left to do is to thread the beads. Collect together 10 or 11 beads; include one larger-diameter bead and cut a length of elastic about 250 mm (10 in) long. Thread it through the beads, putting the one with the larger centre on last. Tie the elastic in a reef knot so that it will not loosen, cut off the surplus elastic and tuck the knot into the large centre bead. Check for size, removing or adding beads where necessary.

Project 4
Bead necklace

To make a paper bead necklace.

Materials required:
- As for making a bracelet, but replace the elastic with strong cotton thread.
- Darning needle
- Clasps (optional)

Procedure

To make necklace of 600 mm (24 in) in length, about 25 beads are required. The paper strips can be approximately 25 mm (1 in) at their widest, and could be longer, making the beads thicker when the paper is rolled. Also it will not matter so much if the beads are not completely symmetrical. In fact you could make some that are tapered, which can be attached to the necklace sideways on (see Figure 3.8).

Make the beads as for the bracelet. Check how much cotton thread is required for the necklace, and thread the darning needle. It is a good idea to lay out the design of the necklace before threading beads on the needle. If you are planning to have

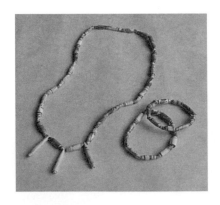

Figure 3.8

some beads endways on, make sure that they are in the right position and that holes have been made to accept the needle. Thread the beads, tie the thread and tuck the knot into a bead. Instead of tying the thread, a clasp could be attached to give the necklace a more professional look.

Papier-mâché

Papier-mâché, although a little messy, can be used for enjoyable craft projects for the elderly. The following projects are best made on a flat surface, and where water and a sink are available.

Newspaper is the long time favourite for making papier-mâché as it gives a stronger finished product. When working with the elderly, I would suggest using paper towel instead of newspaper. It is much cleaner for them to use, and they will not get printing ink on their hands or clothes.

The first project will be to make a small plate, which, when painted and varnished, will make an attractive gift or keepsake.

Project 5
Papier-mâché plate

Making a small plate.

Materials required:
- A small plate to use as a mould
- A saucer
- Newspaper or kitchen towel
- 25-mm household brush
- Bowl for glue (I use a large plastic dog's dish. The size makes it easier for several people to work from)
- PVA glue (wallpaper paste could be used, as long as it is fungicide free)
- (PVA also makes a stronger papier-mâché)
- Petroleum jelly
- Scissors

Procedure

In the dish mix PVA with water at about six parts of water to one of glue.

Cover the table with a sheet of plastic, to catch glue drips. Place the plate that is to be used for the mould on the upturned saucer; this will keep the plate off of the table while it is being worked on. Smear the mould surface (the upturned plate) with a good coating of petroleum jelly. This will make it easier to remove the papier-mâché from the mould.

The paper can now be torn into strips, about 35 mm to 40 mm ($1\frac{1}{4}$ in to $1\frac{1}{2}$ in) wide and a little longer than the diameter of the plate. It is preferable that the strips be torn rather than cut with scissors. I suggest that the paper is folded and then torn on the crease. This will give a ragged edge which, when applied with the glue to the mould, blends together with the other strips better than a cut edge.

Lay strips of paper across the centre of the mould on the petroleum jelly; the ends of the strip should overlap the edge of the mould. These can be cut off later. Lie other strips side by side, until the surface of the mould is completely covered (see Figure 3.9). Apply glue to the strips on the mould, lay more

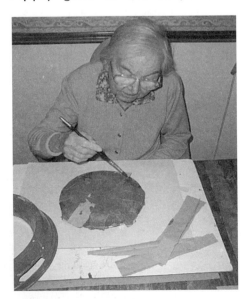

Figure 3.9

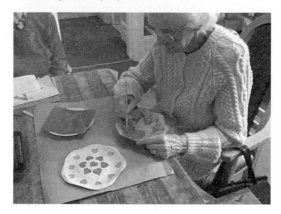

Figure 3.10

strips at 90 degrees to the first ones. Let this layer dry. Add another seven or eight layers of strips in the same manner, alternating the direction of each layer. Make sure that the mould is completely covered each time.

When the paper is completely dry, trim the excess paper from around the edge of the plate. Gently ease the papier mâché off the mould. Wipe off the petroleum jelly with a warm damp sponge, and leave to dry.

The papier-mâché plate can now be shaped, if so desired, and then painted in a base colour; an emulsion household paint will do. When it is dry it can be decorated (see Figure 3.10). To make the plate more durable, two or three coats of varnish can be applied, in matt or gloss finish. Each layer of varnish should be completely dry before applying the next.

Project 6
Papier-mâché bowl

Making an irregular-shaped papier-mâché bowl, using a balloon.

Materials required:
- Same materials as in project 5, except for plate and saucer
- Round balloon

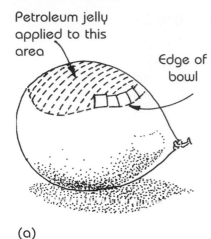

Petroleum jelly applied to this area

Edge of bowl

(a)

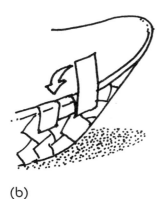

(b)

Figure 3.11

Procedure

Mix up the PVA glue as in the previous project.

Have several sheets of the paper torn into 20 mm to 25 mm ($\frac{3}{4}$ in to 1 in) squares.

Blow up the balloon so that it is a good size and quite hard. Tie securely, as you do not want air to escape. Apply petroleum jelly to an area of the balloon as in Figure 3.11a.

Apply the first layer of paper without glue, attaching the torn paper pieces directly to the petroleum jelly.

Put several pieces of paper squares into the glue dish. They will absorb the glue quite quickly and can be placed onto the balloon in the appropriate area. When transferring the paper pieces from the glue dish to the balloon, rubber gloves could be worn, or kitchen tongs could be used.

Do make sure that the paper pieces form the edge of the bowl with straight edges (see Figure 3.11a). Apply another seven or eight layers of paper, turning and overlapping the pieces at each layer. Brushing more glue on the paper now in place on the balloon will give a good bond when adding more paper.

When the papier-mâché bowl is completely dry, carefully separate the bowl from the balloon. Wipe out the petroleum jelly.

To give a stronger edge to the bowl, glue paper around the edges, turning them into the bowl as shown (see Figure 3.11b).

A solid colour or design can be painted on using acrylic paints. If more durability is desired, varnish with several coats when the paint is dry. Always varnish in a well ventilated room or outdoors.

An alternative to using paper towels in this project is to use different coloured tissue paper. As the tissue paper is somewhat transparent it will give a lively and translucent result. Using only three or four layers will help keep this translucency. The edges could be left ragged to give a natural effect. Take care when removing the papier-mâché as it will be quite delicate. I suggest that the bowl be varnished to make it more rigid.

Other papier-mâché projects appear in chapter 8 on projects for festive occasions.

Decoupage

Decoupage was rediscovered in England during the Victorian era, and became a fashionable pastime. Old greetings cards and clippings from magazines, plus speciality books with ornate coloured motifs, were used to decorate almost anything that had a smooth bare surface.

The following projects make use of tin cans, bottles and show how to build a trinket box and a pen/pencil holder. As metal paint has to be used on the rim and base of the cans, it is advisable that painting and brush cleaning be done in a well ventilated area or outside.

Project 7
Crayon or pen holder

To transform a tin can into a children's crayon or pen holder.

Materials required:
- Clean, empty tin can, to suit size of crayons or pens
- Red or blue metal paint
- Small household brush
- Paint thinners, to clean brush
- PVA glue
- Dish to hold glue
- Scissors (dressmaker's or manicure type)
- Varnish, gloss or matt as desired
- Fine sandpaper
- Old magazines and children's comics

Tips

When using the manicure scissors, the curve of the scissors should be opposite to the curve of the motif being cut.
When cutting a curved shape with scissors, move the item being cut rather than the scissors.

Procedure

Remove label from tin can by immersing the can in warm water. Dry thoroughly.

Most cans have a rim at the top and bottom, which is hard to cover with paper, so I suggest that the tins are painted with metal paint. Make sure that the paint covers the rim on the inside as well as the outside.

The bottom of the can could also be painted to finish it off nicely. Leave the paint to dry overnight.

The can now needs to be covered on the outside completely. From the magazines, have the participant(s) select a colour scheme; it should be fairly plain, as this layer will eventually be partially covered with motifs. The sections of the magazines should be cut into irregular shapes, about 25-mm (1-in) sized pieces.

Mix the PVA glue with water in the dish. You will need a good strength to make the paper stick to the metal. I suggest one part of glue to three parts of water. The glue should now be applied to the part of the can that is to be covered. The glue will run a little, so have a piece of plastic under it to catch the drips. I prefer using plastic here instead of paper, as the glue that drips on the plastic can be wiped up.

The clippings can now be put in position, over-lapping each piece so that the tin does not show. Straight edges butted up to the top and bottom rims of the can will give a nice clean finish. More clippings can be added so that the entire tin is covered; any air bubbles should be smoothed out. The can should now be left to dry. Check for any loose pieces that should be re-glued before proceeding further.

Suitable motifs can be selected from the magazines or comics, depending on the final recipient of the holder. Using the manicure scissors carefully cut out the motifs. It is a good idea to lay out the motifs before gluing, so that a suitable design can be arranged. When a satisfactory design has been decided upon glue motifs in place. The can should be allowed to dry again.

When the motifs are completely dry, varnish can now be applied. This should be done in a well-ventilated room or outdoors. To aid in the varnishing process, the can may be upturned and placed over a bottle, making it easier to rotate while applying varnish. Apply the varnish, brushing in one direction only. Leave it to dry before another coat is applied. Alternate the direction of the brush stroke when each layer of varnish is applied After the fourth coat, when the varnish is totally dry, lightly sand the surface. Apply another 12 to 15 coats of varnish and sand down after every fourth coat. As a final touch, the decoupage could be waxed with white furniture polish.

To complete the project, line the inside with heavy paper. Try the paper in the can and make sure that it overlaps itself by about 20 mm ($\frac{3}{4}$ in). Measure the inside distance of the can from the base to the underside of the rim. Transfer this amount to the paper and cut off the excess. Making it a little undersize will ensure that it fits under the rim. Apply glue to the inside of the can and insert the paper, pushing it against the sides of the can to attach it firmly.

Project 8
Desk tidy

To make a pencil/pen holder from three paper towel cardboard centres.

Materials required:
- 2B pencil
- Masking tape
- Three cardboard centres from paper towel rolls
- Thick cardboard, for base
- Craft knife
- PVA glue
- Container for glue
- Small brush

- Varnish
- Brush for varnishing
- Magazines
- Scissors

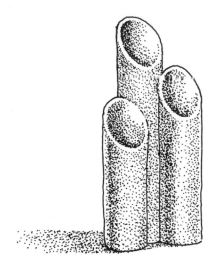

Figure 3.12

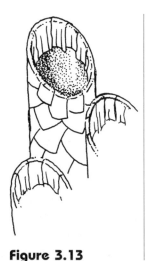

Figure 3.13

Procedure

Using the craft knife, cut the three tubes into three different lengths, 170 mm, 140 mm, and 120 mm ($6\frac{3}{4}$ in, $5\frac{1}{2}$ in, $4\frac{3}{4}$ in). Using scissors, cut the ends of each tube at an angle (see Figure 3.12). Glue them together into the form as shown, using undiluted PVA glue. Let the glue dry. Stand the joined tubes on the thick cardboard and draw a pencil line around the three tubes, transferring the shape onto the cardboard. Make two such shapes and cut them out. These two pieces will be the base of the holder.

Join one of the cardboard bases to the tube assembly, with masking tape. Smooth out any wrinkles in the tape. Feather the tape edges around the tubes by lightly sand papering. Glue the second base onto the first base. This will hide the masking tape and finish off the base bottom.

Cut clippings from the magazines into 20 mm ($\frac{3}{4}$ in) to 25 mm (1 in) pieces.

They can be random shapes. Dilute the glue with more water. The tubes can now be covered with the pieces of paper, each piece being overlapped to cover the cardboard. Straight edges should be used around the bottom of the tubes; make sure that they don't protrude any further.

Clippings can be used to bond the tubes together. The paper needs to be pushed into the joining points of the tubes while still wet.

The clippings should be turned and pasted over the edge and inside the open end of the tubes (see Figure 3.13). A thin lining paper can be inserted in each of the tubes. It should be wide enough so that it just overlaps itself when inserted. Measure it by making it longer than the tube and draw a pencil line around the shape of the open end. The paper can then be removed and the shape cut accurately with scissors. Trim 1 mm ($\frac{1}{16}$ in) off the straight end to ensure that the lining paper sits just below the opening when reinserted. Glue the paper to the inner walls of the tubes.

Twelve to 15 coats of varnish can be applied; sand every fourth layer. Varnish in a well-ventilated room or outdoors.

Project 9
Trinket box

Making a trinket box.

Materials required:
- Corrugated cardboard or thick card (see diagram for size)
- Steel rule
- Craft knife
- 2B Pencil
- PVA glue (wallpaper glue without a fungicide could also be used)
- Magazines
- Varnish
- Brush
- Masking tape
- Small length of wool

Procedure

Refer to Figure 3.14; starting from a square corner of the corrugated cardboard, measure out the pattern for the box as shown. It important that the measuring and cutting is done accurately. This will ensure that the box is square when assembled. Using the craft knife and steel ruler cut out the four corners as indicated. To bend the sides of the box, cut along the dotted line. Cut through one surface of the corrugated board only. Turn the cardboard over and bend up all four sides, securing with tape at the corners. For added strength, tape can be applied to

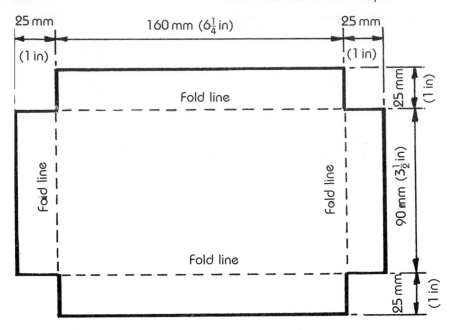

Figure 3.14

the bent edges as well. Place the divider in the box where required and secure with tape. Before attaching the lid, decoupage the inside and outside of the box. I would suggest using fairly neutral colours for the inside, the outside could be bright with a design of your choice. Mix the glue; dilute the PVA glue considerably. Cut the paper into 20 mm ($\frac{3}{4}$ in) to 25 mm (1 in) random shapes. Let these pieces soak in the glue for a while; when saturated they will fold over edges and shape themselves more easily to the corners. Do make sure when applying paper pieces at the corners that they are pushed well in. Avoid creases. The edges of the cardboard should be covered at this time to hide the inside of the corrugated cardboard.

Apply paper pieces to the top of the lid, turning the edges over to the underside. A piece of coloured paper could be used for the underside. Cut it using the steel ruler and craft knife. It should be sized so that it is 1 mm ($\frac{1}{16}$ in) less all round than the lid's dimension. Glue this piece in place and allow it to dry. The lid can now be attached with masking tape. If a more durable hinge is required, duck or book

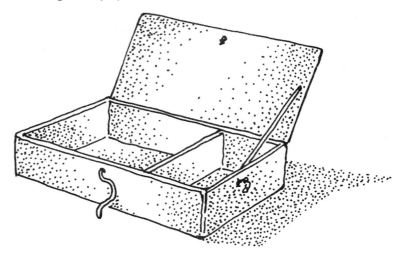

Figure 3.15

binding tape should be used. The tape hinge can be covered paper and finished as the rest of the box, or left if book-binding tape is used.

In a well-ventilated room apply 12 to 15 coats of varnish. Criss-cross each layer and allow the varnish to dry before applying the next. Lightly sand every fourth coat after the varnish is dry. The final coat of varnish should be applied in straight strokes.

A piece of wool or metallic thread can be used to tie the lid closed and to prevent the lid from opening too far. Make a hole in the front of the lid and the box. Knot two short pieces of wool or thread and pass a piece through either hole so that the knots are on the inside. Do the same at the sides but just use one piece of wool. Adjust the length of the wool so that the lid does not open all the way (see Figure 3.15).

Paper flowers

The construction of paper flowers is also covered in chapter 8 (under spring flowers and Easter bonnet decoration). The following will give further ideas for table decoration. Also included is a variation on rose construction.

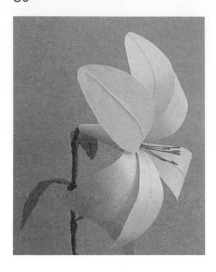

Project 10
Lilies

Materials required:
- White copier paper, A4 size (three sheets required per flower)
- Wire
- Clear adhesive tape
- Masking tape
- Scissors
- Wire cutters
- Green crepe paper
- Glue stick
- Pencil
- PVA glue
- Yellow acrylic paint
- Small round paint brush

Procedure

Making the petals: To construct the lily petals: for one flower you will need three sheets of white paper. Fold the three sheets into quarters. They should now measure 105 mm × 150 mm ($4\frac{1}{8}$ in × $5\frac{3}{4}$ in). Open the first fold only and cut all three sheets along the crease. You should now have six folded (quarter) sheets. Cut six pieces of wire 250 mm (10 in) long. Open up one of the folded papers and position the wire along the centre of one side (see Figure 3.16).

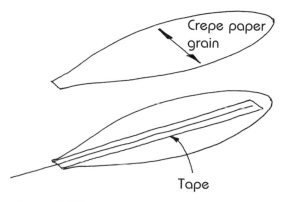

Crepe paper grain

Tape

Figure 3.16

The wire should be as straight as possible. Using the clear tape attach it securely in place. Repeat this procedure for the other five pieces. Apply glue to the insides of the folded papers, making sure that the tape is covered, and stick them together with the wires inside. Make an open template of the lily petal from the pattern section. Centre this over the length of wire and pencil round the template to form the petal shape. Cut out this petal along the pencilled line, turning the paper and not the scissors, to get a clean smooth edge. Curve each slender petal by bending the central wire within. Repeat for the remaining five pieces. Gather the six petals together, and bind the exposed wires with masking tape to hold them together temporarily while you do the next step.

Cut a piece of the thicker wire to 800 mm (32 in) and bend it double to strengthen it. Insert one end into the exposed wires of the blossom and secure with masking tape. Cut 20 mm ($\frac{3}{4}$ in) strips of the crepe paper and wind it around the wire, starting about 50 mm (2 in) from the base of the petals. The cone shape which forms the base of the petals can be made from the same copier paper, or if you have some white card, use this instead. The copier paper does tend to crinkle a little when wrapping it into a cone. Cut a piece 105 mm × 150 mm ($4\frac{1}{8}$ in × $5\frac{3}{4}$ in). Before attaching it to the flower, roll the paper diagonally to form a cone. Trim off the pointed corner at the wide end. Cut this off so that the wide end of the cone is straight. Now unroll it and place it at the base of the blossom, wrapping it around the wires to form a cone again. Push the wide end well onto the petal base. Glue the cone to itself to prevent it unwrapping. The green crepe paper should emerge from the small end of the cone. Arrange the petals to form the natural shape of a lily blossom. Bend the wire at the small end of the cone; it should be at an angle of about 90 degrees.

Making the stamen: Using the fine wire cut six lengths 70 mm ($2\frac{3}{4}$ in) long. Cut six pieces of masking tape about 8 mm ($\frac{1}{4}$ in) wide 25 mm (1 in) long. Wrap the tape at the end of each piece of wire. Using masking tape, tape all six pieces together, at the other end. The stamen can be painted yellow and left to dry. When dry glue in place.

Making leaves: Cut six rectangle shapes of green crepe paper 120 mm × 40 mm (4$\frac{3}{4}$ in × 1$\frac{1}{2}$ in). The grain should run crosswise to the length of the leaf. Cut six pieces of thin wire to 180 mm (7 in). Make sure the wire is straight and lay a piece lengthways along the centre of a piece of crepe paper. Attach securely with a strip of clear tape along the full length of wire. Repeat for the other five pieces. Using the leaf pattern cut out the shape. Attach the leaves to the main stem with the wire on the underside, using masking tape. Bend the wire to give a natural leaf shape. The stem can be wrapped with crepe paper or florist's tape to complete the flower.

Lilies can have more than one flower on each stem. If you decide to add more, strengthen the stem with additional or thicker wire. For a more natural looking blossom try using watercolour paper, instead of copier paper. With the paper moistened and with watercolour pigments, delicate shades of yellows and greens could then be painted on.

Project 11
Roses

Materials required:
- Crepe paper – green, red, yellow or orange
- Florist's tape (optional)
- Thick and thin wire
- PVA glue
- Glue stick
- Wire cutters
- Pencil
- Adhesive tape
- Cotton wool

Procedure

For one rose cut the following petals forms from the pattern section of the book: five of No 1, three of No 2, five of No 2 and three of No 4. Cut a piece of wire 300 mm (12 in) long. The grain should be running across the petal. Smooth and stretch the crepe paper by gently pulling between the thumb and first finger. Shape the petals by rolling around a pencil (see Figure 3.17). Cut several leaf shapes.

Dab a little glue on the end of the wire and wrap a No 1 petal around the wire. Add more glue and wrap the remaining four petals, alternating their position each time. Apply a small amount of glue at the base of the petal only. Colour in crepe paper bleeds easily if it gets too moist.

Attach all the remaining petals in the same manner. Shape the outer edges of the petals as you build the rose. The calyx can now be glued in position using the glue stick

The leaves can be strengthened by attaching a piece of thin wire to the underside with clear adhesive tape. Leave enough wire protruding to attach to others, making groups of threes. It is also necessary to have enough wire to attach to the main stem. Tape is used to hold the leaf assemblies to the main stem. Any exposed wire should be wrapped with florist's tape or thin strips of green crepe paper.

To make a rose bud, cut a piece of wire to the desired length. This will depend on whether it is to be attached to the main stem or used separately. Make one end into a hook and glue a small ball of

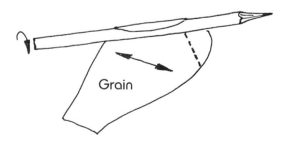

Grain

Figure 3.17

cotton wool to it. Wrap the wool with the crepe paper of your chosen colour for the bud. Use a small piece of adhesive tape to secure it. Cut a size 3 petal and wrap it around the bud base. Apply the petal at an angle so that it wraps and tapers nicely like a rosebud. Only a small dot of glue should be used to hold it in position. To make the calyx cut a 80-mm (3-in) circle from the green crepe paper. Cut this into a five-pointed star. Push the calyx onto the wire and up to the rosebud, attaching it with the glue stick. Leaves could be added if you wish and the exposed wire wrapped, as in the rose stem example.

Project 12
Poppies

Material required:
- Crepe paper, red, green
- Florist's tape (optional)
- Copier paper
- Thick wire
- Pliers with cutting edge
- Scissors
- Pencil
- PVA glue
- Toothpick
- Cotton wool
- Watercolour paints, red and blue
- Small brush

Procedure

Without unfolding it, cut a 100-mm (4-in) strip off the full width 390 mm (15 in) of the crepe paper. Fold the strip into thirds and then in half again. Make a poppy template (see the pattern section). Place it on the folded crepe paper and draw the poppy petal shape. Cut out the poppy petals. Cut a piece of wire about 250 mm (10 in) long and bend one end into a hook. To make the centre of the poppy, glue a small ball of cotton wool to the hook

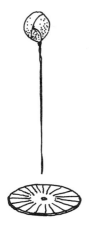

Figure 3.18

end of the wire. Cover with a small circle of the crepe paper and glue in position. Cut a 50-mm (2-in) diameter circle from the copier paper. Mix a dark purple using the watercolours. Paint the poppy centre and both sides of the paper disc. When dry cut slits around the periphery of the disc to almost reach the centre. Carefully make a hole at the disc centre and push it onto the straight end of wire stem up to the cotton wool bud (see Figure 3.18). Glue in position.

Smooth and stretch six petals carefully between the thumb and first finger. Roll the edges over a pencil as described in the previous project. Attach the petals to the underside of the poppy centre, gluing at the petal base. Add the remaining petals at various intervals around the base. Shape the petals to a natural form. The exposed wire can be wrapped with green crepe paper or florist's tape.

Chapter 4

Modelling with clay, Plasticine and salt dough

Modelling with clay
Modelling Plasticine
Modelling using synthetic modelling material
Modelling with salt dough

Modelling with any form of elastic material has a very healing aspect. Art therapists recommend modelling to those suffering from depression and other disturbed states of mind. These media can be introduced to older people without them feeling they need to have had any art training. The projects I have included in this chapter are very basic and can be accomplished fairly easily. More complex details can be added to the completed pieces if the participant can manage detailed work.

There are many modelling materials now available. Clay, Plasticine and salt dough are the modelling media that I use mainly. I have also included in this chapter modelling with a synthetic medium that can be hardened in an oven.

Each of the modelling media that will be explained in this chapter requires different working techniques. These techniques will give people the opportunity of seeing how the different materials respond to their touch.

Plasticine is clean to work with, does not dry out and it requires very little preparation. I use it quite often in my activities programme, as it can be brought out as an interim activity if someone is in need of a change of project.

Modelling with clay

Clay, although requiring more preparation, gives greater possibilities, especially for hand-building projects. This is an ideal material for larger forms. I also think that it is a good substance for older people to experience and work with, since many of them may not have had the chance to do so in their youth.

One of the women in a group I worked with was very keen to make a swan. I gave her a piece of clay and without any help, and within a few minutes, she had formed a very good likeness of a swan.

I will often work alongside a person, and show how easy it is to make a simple object like a mouse, a hedgehog or even a larger animal. The form is created by shaping, pressing and gently squeezing the clay. It is always preferable that the shape be created from the whole piece, rather than trying to add pieces such as legs or tails.

Clay work does require a few special tools – wire for cutting the clay and some modelling tools. However, if you do not want to buy special equipment, the kitchen drawer is a good source of some helpful implements (see Figure 4.1). As the projects all use hand-building techniques, rolling guides are extremely useful for producing slabs of equal thickness. They can be made from pieces of wood, 5 mm ($\frac{1}{4}$ in) thick. When rolling slabs of any elastic substance, the guides are placed either side with the rolling pin straddling them. The clay can then be rolled to a uniform thickness.

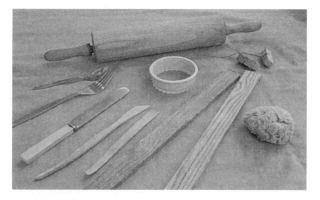

Figure 4.1

A potter's wheel is not necessary. Glazing and firing are not dealt with here; instead, I suggest that the clay be painted when dry. A point that must be remembered is that if finished work is left unsealed, it will absorb moisture. If immersed in water for long enough it will dissolve. This can be an advantage at those times when you want to reuse clay from discarded or broken forms.

A work board is desirable. Thick plywood of a size about 300 mm × 400 mm (12 in × 16 in) is recommended. The board should be covered with hessian, which is stapled securely to the back. This will prevent the clay from sticking to the surface.

Clay is available in 25-kg bags from potteries or ceramic suppliers and is usually in a good malleable state, ready for working. It will keep for an indefinite period as long as it is not allowed to dry out, when it becomes unworkable. Clay that has dried out completely can be reconstituted by immersing it in water for a period of time. To rectify clay that is just a little dry, wrap it in a heavy damp cloth (smaller clay pieces will absorb the water more quickly) and seal it in a plastic bag. A bucket with a lid is a useful storage facility. Keep it in a cool place, with a damp cloth and piece of plastic over the top. It is quite possible that mould will grow on the clay if kept in a warm place. This will not harm it in any way and can be rinsed off.

Before working with clay it should be prepared or wedged. Put the clay onto the board and, using the cutting wire, slice off a piece about the size of a small loaf of bread. Put the excess back into the plastic bag. With both hands, knead the clay thoroughly, just as you would when making bread, except that this process is to *expel* any air that might be trapped in the clay. A potter's nightmare is air trapped in a piece that is fired. Air bubbles, expanding in the heat, can cause the clay to explode or crack in the kiln. Kneading is not so important for the projects in this book, as they are not to be fired. It will, however, make the clay more homogeneous and pliable, something that mature hands will be grateful for. It is a good idea to use a moisturising cream after working with clay and washing hands.

Completed solid clay objects when drying are prone to cracking. To avoid this, hollow out the inside a little. Wrapping clay objects loosely in plastic will also slow the drying process and help to prevent cracking.

Project 1
Thumb pot

Making a thumb pot using earthenware clay.

Materials required:
- Earthenware clay
- Thin wire for cutting clay
- Work board
- Modelling tools or dinner knife and spoon
- Acrylic paint
- Brush
- Varnish

Procedure

Cut a piece of clay, and wedge it as described above. Cut from this a small piece that fits comfortably in the palm of the hand.

Make the piece of clay into a smooth ball, as round as possible, by rotating it in the hands. Once this has been done, hold the ball of clay in the palm of one hand. Using the thumb of the other hand, start pressing it inwards bit by bit, towards the centre of the clay, rotating the clay as you do so. By pressing the thumb towards the fingers of the right hand, the hole will begin to enlarge. Continue rotating with a gentle even pressure all the way round, until the desired shape is reached (see Figure 4.2). As the clay is pressed further it will get thinner and larger. It can now be easily formed into a dish. The edges could then be scalloped and some decoration added (see Figure 4.3). It will be obvious that a variety of shapes

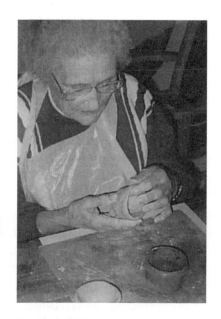

Figure 4.2

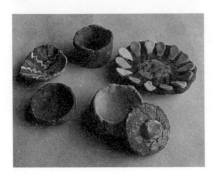

Figure 4.3

can be formed using this simple procedure. One word of warning: do not let the clay wall get too thin. Thin clay, when dried, becomes very fragile. It is also important that the clay is of fairly even thickness throughout. Tools can be used to shape and smooth the pot as required.

The thumb pot can be left to dry. When it is completely dry it can be painted with acrylic paint and varnished, if so wished.

The following projects involve joining clay pieces together. If the finished work is to be glazed and fired, clay should be joined together with slip to give a stronger joint. Slip is clay in a more liquid state, and it is often also used for decorating the finished piece. There are many books specializing in clay work that will give more suggestions on finishing. I have simplified the process of this project so that the completed item is to be painted rather than glazed and fired. If you have access to a kiln and wish to have the finished product fired, I suggest that you get further advice on glazing and firing as it is quite a specialized procedure.

Project 2
Coil pot

Building a coil pot.

Materials required:
- Earthenware clay
- Thin wire for cutting clay
- Work board
- Modelling tools or dinner knife and spoon
- Dish with water
- Rolling pin
- 2 rolling guides (sticks)
- Round biscuit cutter or jam jar, about 70 mm to 80 mm in diameter
- Acrylic paint
- Brush
- Varnish

- Plastic bags
- Small piece of paper or card

Procedure

Cut about a 130 mm (5 in) cube of clay and wedge it thoroughly. Cut off a section, a little larger than the cutter or jam jar; the base of the pot will be cut from this piece. Place this clay on the work board and press it so that it is reasonably flat. Arrange the rolling guides either side of the clay and position the rolling pin on them (see Figure 4.4). Roll the clay so that it becomes the thickness of the guides. It should be a uniform thickness. With the cutter or jam jar, cut out a circle of clay. (The remainder can be wedged in with the remaining clay later.)

Ease the circle of clay off the board with the knife and place it back down onto a circle of paper or card. This process makes it easier for the finished pot to be removed from the board later, and enables the pot to be freely turned as the coils are pressed down.

Cut several small pieces of clay and roll them into lengths of coil using the fingers of both hands (see Figure 4.5). They should finish up about 8 mm ($\frac{1}{4}$ in) in diameter. The rolling should be done fairly quickly so the clay does not dry out. If the coil becomes too

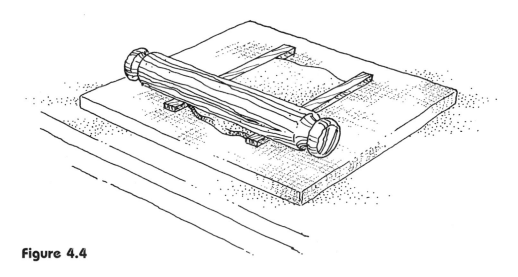

Figure 4.4

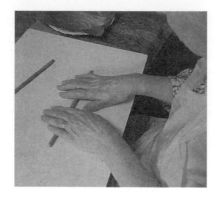

Figure 4.5

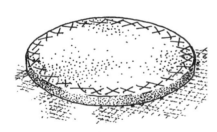

(a)

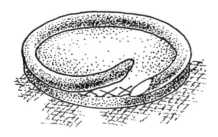

(b)

Figure 4.6

long and unwieldy cut the coil down to a manageable length. The coils can be joined when building the pot. It is important to keep the diameter of the coils consistent throughout their length. Some difficulty may be experienced in this process, as there is a tendency to press too hard. The coil then becomes flat and will not roll. An even, light pressure should be maintained, using a forward and backward motion and just the length of the fingers for the complete roll.

As mentioned, it is important that the clay does not dry out, which can happen quite quickly in a warm environment. Also, older people do not work very quickly. Place clay and coils in a plastic bag, or cover them over, to slow the drying process.

Now that some coils have been made, the next step is to start joining them to the base. Using the wood modelling tool, lightly score the clay around the edge of the base and a piece of the clay coil (see Figure 4.6a). Dip your finger in the water and moisten the scored edge and coil. The clay should be well moistened before attaching the coil to the base. Press the coil into the base with the thumb, supporting the outside wall with the other hand. When joining coils lengthways, cut the ends at an angle as shown in Figure 4.6b and moisten the ends before joining. The first coil should be attached completely around the base before adding another row.

The shape of the pot has to be considered before adding more coils. In this particular case, the pot's circumference is to increase for two coils and then reduce. When attaching the next coil, score and moisten as before and place the coil to *the outer edge* of the first coil. Gently press down with the thumb all the way around each new coil. When pressing the coils, support them with the other hand. This is very important when using the coil method to build large pots. Add another row in the same manner, placing the coil at the outer edge. The next coil should be placed on the inside edge so that the circumference of the pot begins to get smaller; another coil is then applied to the inside edge to

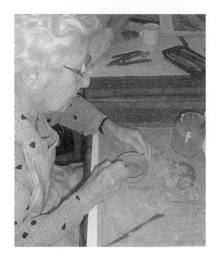

decrease the circumference further. A final coil can now be attached to make the rim of the pot. This is placed a little to the outside edge of the last coil, completing the pot's contour.

The pot can be left with the coils showing, or they can be joined together by smoothing. Use a finger or flat tool to pull the coils together, hiding the joints. When blending on the inside of the pot, again support the walls by cradling the outside of the pot with the other hand. The surface can be smoothed with the hand or a damp sponge. When the pot has dried a little more the outer surface can be burnished with the back of a spoon. This gives it an attractive polished surface. While the pot is at this hardened stage, or what is termed 'leather hard,' a design can be inscribed into the surface with a sharp tool. The person's initials can be scratched onto the base at this time also. Any pointed tool will do.

When the clay has dried completely, it can be decorated, using acrylic paint. Unfired clay is a porous substance so you may have to give it several coats of paint; you could also paint the entire pot with a base colour first, and then add a design when dry. If the pot is left unpainted or un-sealed it is susceptible to moisture; it will break down to its natural state when immersed in water.

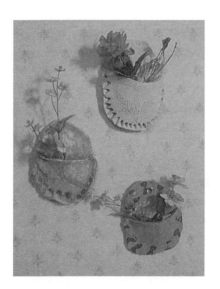

Project 3
Wall plaque

Constructing a wall plaque.

Materials required:
- Pottery tools as for project 2
- Dried flowers or twigs
- Sheet of newspaper

Procedure

Cut a piece of clay about the size of a large grape-fruit. Wedge it a little as described previously. Cut

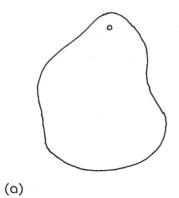

(a)

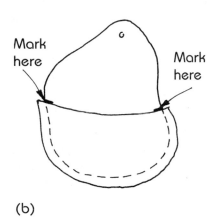

Mark
here

Mark
here

(b)

Figure 4.7

this again so that one piece is larger than the other. Take the larger piece and press it reasonably flat on the work board, it should still be a little thicker than the rolling guides. Place the guides either side of the clay and roll it flat, at an even thickness, using the rolling pin. Make sure that the rolling pin straddles the rolling guides. This piece will be for the back of the plaque. Cut out the shape similar to the one in Figure 4.7a. Set it aside for a moment.

The smaller piece of clay, which will be the pocket, can now be rolled, using the same procedure as the first piece. It needs to be a shape similar to that shown but a little larger so that it will overhang (see Figure 4.7b). Lie the dried twig or flower on top of the pocket piece and roll it into the clay using the rolling pin. A light pressure is all that is required. Lift the twig out of the clay when you have rolled in all the dried twig or flower shapes desired. To attach the pocket, crumple up a small piece of the newspaper and lay it in position on the back piece. Lay the pocket piece in its correct place over the newspaper to form a pocket – it should overhang the back piece. Carefully cut off this overhang, following the shape of the back. On the back piece mark the location of the pocket (see Figure 4.7b). You will then be able to replace it in the exact position. Remove the pocket and turn it over. Score the edges lightly with a tool, but only where the joint will be. Score the edges of the back piece, just to the marks that you made. Moisten both scored areas liberally. With the newspaper ball still in position, realign the pocket on the back form, lining up the edges of both the forms. Press the two pieces together with your thumb or a tool, making sure that they are well joined.

A hanging hole now needs to be made; the blunt end of a pencil can be used to make the hole. Press it firmly through the clay. Do not put it too close to the edge, as it will weaken the edge at that point.

With a knife, gently ease the completed plaque off of the work board, and place it on another board or tray to dry.

Modelling with Plasticine

Make sure that the Plasticine is pliable before putting it to use. It can be hard for older people to model with Plasticine when it is cold and hard. Warm it in your hands, or leave it on a radiator for a few minutes. Older people may reject this material initially as they may think they are being given childish projects. Plasticine, however, has a wide variety of uses, especially as it is available in several colours. It can be used to try out a design that can be built later in clay or salt dough. It is ideal for producing a papier-mâché mould, or just to explore three-dimensional forms. Whatever the project, it is an excellent modelling material for revitalising mature hands.

I sometimes start a modelling activity by giving a warmed, golf ball-size piece of Plasticine to a resident, and let him or her roll and shape it in his or her hands. It is very interesting to watch as a form is created – usually a human or animal shape evolves. People may need a bit of encouragement if they have problems modelling a recognizable object; I tell them it does not matter what it turns out to be. Any shape can be interesting enough; just using their hands is the important point of this activity.

I find it a good plan, when starting people on new projects, to work alongside them. If a particular shape is the goal, then I show them what the rough shape should look like to begin with, using another piece of Plasticine.

Project 4
Hedgehogs and others

Making simple Plasticine forms.

Materials required:
- Plasticine, any colour will do
- Work board
- Knife
- Modelling tool
- Knitting needle

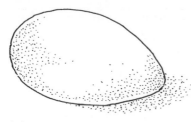

(a)

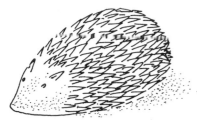

(b)

Figure 4.8

If you are assisting someone, cut two pieces of Plasticine, about the size of a golf ball, warm them in your hands or on a radiator. Suggest that you both are going to make a hedgehog (see Figure 4.8).

Start by making a ball from the Plasticine, rolling it in the palm of your hands. Taking the ball in your hand, work it into an egg shape (Figure 4.8a). Use the thumb and first finger to smooth the shape until it resembles a pointed egg shape, similar to a hedgehog form. Tap the form on the work board to flatten the underside.

Starting a little back from the snout, use the tool to create spiky hair. The eyes can be now be put in using the point of the knitting needle and thus completing the hedgehog (Figure 4.8b).

Try a mouse next. It is the same procedure as the hedgehog. Create a ball and then an egg shape. The nose should be more pointed than in the hedgehog. Now flatten it as before.

When modelling any material it is better to shape appendages like tails and ears by pressing and shaping, rather than by adding pieces. To create a tail, start gathering and pulling the Plasticine out, thinning it until it is at the required length and thickness. Smooth areas of the body that may require it, with the finger and thumb. Turn the form so that you are looking down the nose to the tail and pinch out some ears. Add the eyes, as with the hedgehog.

Try the other forms as shown. Remember to add legs, wings, etc., by pulling and pinching and not by adding pieces.

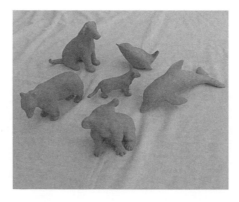

Project 5
Rose centrepiece

Making a rose centrepiece.

Materials required:
- Plasticine, colours – red, yellow and green
- Shallow tin, painted or decoupaged
- Wire

Procedure

Decide which colour Plasticine to use for the rose and cut off a piece about the size of a marble. Roll this into a ball between the palms of your hands. With the ball between the thumb and first finger, start pressing the Plasticine. Continue applying pressure and turning the form until it becomes a flat circle. As this and subsequent forms are going to be the petals, they need to be as thin as possible. When you are satisfied that the Plasticine is thin enough, put it down on the work board, pick up an edge and roll it up loosely. This piece will be the rose centre (see Figure 4.9). Refer to this figure when making the petals. Start with two more pieces of Plasticine, about the same size as the centre, and roll them into a ball. Flatten each ball into the petal shape. They should be as thin as possible to give the impression of rose petals. Attach the base of the petal to the centre of the rose by using a little pressure, The top of the centre should be in line with the top of the petal. Pull the top of the petal a little away from the centre piece.

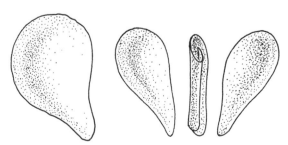

Figure 4.9

The next petals need to be larger. Cut two pieces of Plasticine a little larger than the previous ones. Make the petals as before and attach to base of the centre; overlap the joins of the previous petals. Bend the top of the petals away from the centre to make the rose as natural looking as possible.

Continue making and attaching larger petals until the rose is as large as you would like it. If the base of the rose becomes bulky, trim off the excess with a knife. Insert a piece of wire for the stem.

Make another rose a little smaller with the same colour Plasticine. Using the other colour make another rose, the same as the first. A small bud could also be incorporated in the arrangement. A few leaves should now be made, using the green Plasticine. Refer to Figure 4.10 for the leaf shapes. Assemble the roses and leaves in the container.

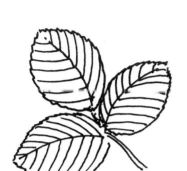

Figure 4.10

Modelling using synthetic modelling material

Synthetic modelling material is available from art materials suppliers and is produced in many colours. It is used in much the same way as Plasticine, with the exception that it can be hardened by baking in an oven. Once hardened it can be carved, sawn, filed and polished. It can be also be painted using acrylic paint.

As long as the material is not hardened it can be reused many times. It can be marbled by mixing with other colours, to obtain a unique colour combination. By kneading the colours together more thoroughly, a uniform colour can be achieved.

Project 6
Marbled beads

Making marbled beads.

Materials required:
- Synthetic modelling material, two colours of your choice

- Smallest size knitting needle
- Glass sheet
- Craft knife
- Rolling pin or bottle

Procedure

Cut two pieces of equal size from either colour. Roll each piece into a thin sausage. Twist together like a candy cane and knead until you have the desired marbling effect. Roll into a sausage again keeping a circular form throughout. Continue rolling until you have the size of bead that you require. Cut small pieces off the roll, and make each piece into a ball by rolling it in the palm of your hands. Flatten with a rolling pin, and make the hole with the knitting needle. If you require an even thickness use rolling guides when rolling out (as explained in the clay work projects). Harden in an oven using the recommended temperature setting.

The following project will need good eyesight and nimble fingers, but it will show how simple it is to make unique jewellery.

Project 7
Leaf brooch

A leaf brooch.

Materials required:
- Synthetic modelling material, dark olive
- Small semiprecious stone
- Rolling pin or bottle
- Small leaf with a good vein structure
- Clasp finding
- Bonding glue
- Craft knife

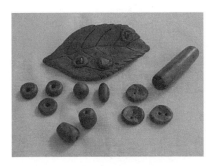

Procedure

Depending on the size of leaf cut a piece of the modelling material to suit. Knead thoroughly and roll it to about 5 mm ($\frac{1}{4}$ in) thick. Lay the leaf on the modelling material and lightly roll leaf into the material. Cut out the leaf shape and remove the leaf. The leaf veins should be impressed in the modelling material. If it is not to your satisfaction, start the process over again. Re-knead so that it is warm and roll out as before. Roll the leaf in with more pressure this time.

To add the decorative stone, roll out very thin coils about 2 mm ($\frac{1}{16}$ in) in diameter. Place the stone in position and press it into the leaf design. Wrap the thin coil around the stone, pressing it carefully so that it bonds with the rest of the material and also supports the stone. Thin coils can be made into additional decorative embellishments.

Small stones are set in the material by rolling small balls of modelling material, placing them on the design in the desired position and pushing a stone into each ball.

The material is hardened in an oven making sure to use the manufacturer's temperature setting and hardening time.

A clasp can be attached to the back with a strong bonding glue after it has been hardened.

Modelling with salt dough

This form of modelling goes back to ancient Egyptian times, if not earlier. Almost every country has used this process to create figurines for religious festivals. It is used in many countries for the creation of decorative objects, and can be seen at craft markets throughout the British Isles.

The dough is made from regular plain white flour, salt and water. When dried or baked, the completed objects can be decorated in brightly coloured designs to give them a festive look. Water-based paints such as watercolours, gouache or acrylic can be used. Dough can also be coloured during the mixing process using food colouring. The completed pieces can be made more durable with the application of oil-based varnish. Dough art is ideal for making gifts, keepsakes and festival ornaments, as well as for functional pieces.

There are several different recipes for salt dough. Various proportions of the ingredients will give different strengths. The following recipe will give dough that has a good strength, suitable for standing figures. The quantities shown make enough dough for several projects. If you have dough left over, seal it in a plastic bag and refrigerate. It will keep for several days.

Standard salt dough recipe

16 oz (2 cups) flour, 16 oz (2 cups) salt plus water. The amount of water will depend on the consistency required.

Mix the flour and salt together in the mixing bowl, add water gradually, sprinkle in drops until the mixture is neither crumbly nor so sticky that it sticks to your hands. Put the dough onto the work board, which should be lightly floured. Knead the dough for 10 to 12 minutes, until it begins to get warm.

Dough art can be dried in the oven, or left to air dry on a radiator. Put the completed pieces on a baking tray when drying. If you dry them in an oven, a low temperature is recommended to avoid cracking. A suggested temperature is 150°C for a period of $2\frac{1}{2}$ hours.

Dough art, before it has an application of paint, looks very much like the real thing, shortbread biscuits, a tempting morsel for the unwary! Do keep them out of reach, as they are not to be eaten.

Dried dough art can be repaired and joined with a dough paste. The dough paste is prepared by mixing a small amount of dough with water until it has a creamy consistency.

Project 8
Egg cup

Making and decorating an egg cup.

Materials required:
- Plain white flour
- Work board
- Dinner knife
- Paint
- Varnish

Procedure

Cut a piece of dough about the size of a tennis ball, and put the remaining dough back in the mixing bowl, covered, so that it does not dry out.

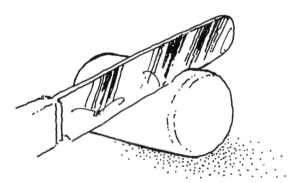

Figure 4.11

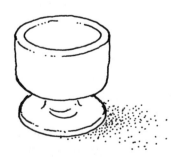

Figure 4.12

Roll the piece of dough back and forth on the work board. Stop rolling when it is about 35 mm in diameter. Cut one end off as evenly as possible (see Figure 4.11). Holding the dough roll in one hand press the thumb of the other hand into the centre of the cut round. Continue pressing with the thumb and turning the dough until the cup for the egg is formed. The inside diameter of an average egg cup is 40 mm ($1\frac{5}{8}$ in) and the inside height is between 30 mm and 40 mm ($1\frac{1}{8}$ in and $1\frac{5}{8}$ in). Once you have the cup formed, start modelling the base, squeezing the dough in to form the neck. Refer to Figure 4.12 for the completed shape.

Follow the recommended drying procedure at the beginning of this section. When the salt dough is completely dry the egg cup can be decorated with a bright design and varnished.

Project 9
Ornamental bowl

Making an ornamental bowl.

Materials required:
- All materials as in project 6 plus the following items
- Two rolling guides about 8 mm ($\frac{1}{4}$ in) thick
- Small basin
- Plastic food wrap

Procedure

Make the dough according to the recipe preceding project 6. Cut a piece of dough about the size of a grapefruit. Roll it to a thickness of about 8 mm ($\frac{1}{4}$ in). Use the rolling guides either side of the dough to get a uniform thickness. The rolled shape should be roughly circular.

Place a piece of food wrap over the upturned basin, this will prevent the dough from sticking to the basin. Carefully lay the rolled dough over the basin. Use your hands to form the dough into the shape of the basin. Cut the scallop design with a knife (see Figure 4.13). Leave the dough on the upturned basin to dry a little. Remove when the dough is dry to the touch. It can then be oven-dried as recommended in the basic instruction before project 6. When dry, decorate with acrylic paint and varnish if required.

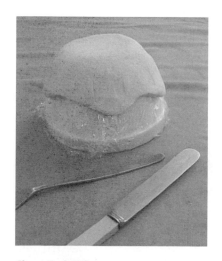

Figure 4.13

Project 10
Napkin rings

Making four napkin rings.

Materials required:
- Salt dough
- Work board
- Rolling pin
- Two rolling guides
- Knife
- Ruler
- Two core tubes of kitchen paper towel
- Small dish for water
- Four dessert spoons

Procedure

Cut the core tubes in half, so that you have four tubes. Pour a little water in the dish. Knead the dough for about 10 minutes, until warm. Flour the work board and roll the dough between the rolling guides, to get an even thickness and an oblong shape. Using the ruler as a straight edge, trim off one end. Cut four strips 40 mm ($1\frac{5}{8}$ in) wide by 200 mm ($7\frac{5}{8}$ in) long. Place a tube on a strip of dough and roll up the dough on the tube. When the dough starts to overlap itself, it should be joined by moistening with a little water. Overlap about 20 mm ($\frac{3}{4}$ in). Refer to Figure 4.14 and support the extended dough piece over the spoon as shown. Make the other rings in the same way.

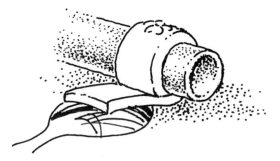

Figure 4.14

Allow them to air dry until the rings hold their shape unsupported. Remove the spoon and tube. Dry as recommended in the basic instructions before project 6. After the drying process, the rings can be decorated with paint and varnished if desired.

Project 11
Picture frame

Decorative   100 mm × 150 mm   (4 in × 6 in) picture frame.

Materials required:
- Dough, see recipe preceding project 6
- Work board
- Rolling pin
- Two rolling guides, 9 mm ($\frac{5}{16}$ in) thick
- Dish of water
- Dinner knife
- Pencil
- Ruler
- Craft knife
- Picture frame template (see pattern section)
- Corrugated cardboard
- Glass, 2 mm × 100 mm × 150 mm ($\frac{3}{64}$ in × 4 in × 6 in)
- Varnish
- Acrylic paint, colours as required
- Brush, small household
- Brushes for acrylic paint

Procedure

Refer to the picture frame information in the pattern section at the end of the book. The size shown is half full size. Using this information draw the shapes on the corrugated cardboard. Cut out all the components. These can be used to mark out the dough to the correct size.

Mix $1\frac{1}{2}$ times the amount of dough shown in the standard recipe. Knead until warm and pliable. Roll the dough using the rolling guides until it is equal in thickness to the guides. As it is not advisable to move the cut components until they are dry, roll the dough where it can be cut and left to dry.

Lay the front frame templates on the dough and lightly mark out the profile with the knife. Remove the template and cut out the frame and window, using the knife and ruler. Remove the excess dough and knead together. Roll out the dough as before, lay the other templates on the dough, mark and cut them out. The excess dough can be put in a plastic bag and refrigerated.

Leave the frame components to dry slowly. Excessive drying heat will cause the items to distort and crack.

When the items are dry they can be joined together. Mix a little dough paste and assemble the components. First attach the three spacing strips. They should be attached a little away from the window cutout (see pattern). Check to see that the photograph and glass will fit easily. There may be a little shrinkage as the dough dries, so do allow for this. Apply the paste to both surfaces and affix using a little pressure. Leave to dry.

When completely dry attach the backing piece in the same way. This should be allowed to dry before attaching the two supports. These should be attached so that the open end will be at the top when the frame is standing. Ensure that the supports have bonded well before standing the frame. Insert glass and photograph.

Embellishments such as leaves, scrolls, flowers, etc. can be added at this stage. When the frame is totally dry, decorate with paint and varnish.

Embellishments

The appeals of dough art are the endless possibilities of adding decorations to completed forms. They can be easily attached using dough paste.

The following project shows how to make rose decorations. The size of the roses will depend on their application and how nimble the fingers are, so adjust as necessary. You may have to consider making these yourself, and have the person you are working with paint them. The process is the same as shown in Plasticine modelling.

Project 12
Decorative roses

Making roses for decoration.

Materials required:
- Dough, amount will depend on size of rose and how many are required
- Rolling pin
- Work board
- Knife
- Dish of water
- Acrylic paint
- Brush
- Varnish
- Brush, household

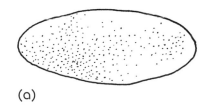

(a)

(b)

Figure 4.15

Procedure

Start with a small amount of dough, about the size of a golf ball. Cut a piece off and roll it flat. Make the shape as show in Figure 4.15a. It needs to be made as thin as possible. Gently press it between the thumb and first finger to get the desired thickness. Roll it up, applying a little water, so that it sticks to itself. This will be the rose centre (Figure 4.15b). Set aside.

Pull off a little more dough and form into two small balls. Press them flat by pressing and turning between the thumb and first finger. The completed rose will look more realistic if these 'petals' are made as thin as possible. Attach with a little water to opposite sides of the rose centre. They can be shaped a little by pulling the top edge away from the centre. Support the rose between two pieces of rolled paper.

Make two more 'petals', but a little larger. Attach and shape and set aside using the support.

More petals can be added, depending on the size required. Air dry using a support to keep their shape. When dry, they can be baked. Finish by painting and varnishing if required.

Chapter 5

Weaving

It has been my experience that older women generally enjoy working with their hands, and weaving is a favourite. I'm sure that the feel of wool brings back fond memories of knitting jumpers, socks and gloves. One woman in my group really enjoys winding wool. She makes tidy balls from skeins and wool oddments contributed to the home. If knitting or crochet work is too difficult because of poor eyesight or hand coordination, weaving on the loom is a possible alternative. Men, too, can be gently persuaded to try their hand at weaving. As older people, especially those with dementia, are apt to forget what to do next, supervision is usually required throughout the weaving process.

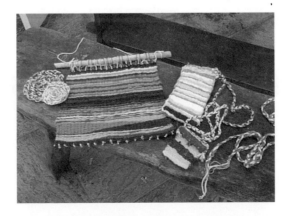

A simple loom can be made from a polystyrene tray, previously used for pre-packed food. As this type of loom is so lightweight, it is ideal for those confined to bed. If a special activities area or room is not available, a lounge setting is suitable for a weaving activity as the work can be done on a person's lap.

I have included working only with a frame loom in this chapter, as it is portable, easy to construct and simple to use. There are, of course, many other types of looms available, which would require a complete book to describe.

The frame loom can be any size or shape, used flat, propped at an angle or even used vertically. The weaving process is relatively slow and the size of the weaving is limited to the size to the frame. None the less, colourful and interesting wall hangings, as well as smaller articles like purses or shoulder bags, can easily be made. These articles make ideal gifts, and are very saleable at fund-raising events.

For those without any weaving experience, the terminology used can be a little complex. However, as the frame loom has very few components, the weaving terms used in the following projects are minimal.

Weaving terminology

Wool yarn that is secured vertically on the frame, is called the 'warp'. Yarn that is interlaced through the warp is called 'weft'. 'Shed' is the opening between the warp threads through which the shuttle is passed. The 'shuttle' is the tool used to pass the weft through the warp. 'Beating' is the term used for packing the weft threads tightly to one another.

As odd balls of wool can be used for the warp and weft, the cost of producing a weaving can be relatively low. Excellent sources of wool can be relatives, friends or church bazaars. It is important, however, to select warp thread with care. It should be quite strong, as it will be under a lot of tension. It should also be quite smooth to allow the shuttle to pass through easily.

I find it very interesting to see the vast differences in the colour schemes chosen by the residents. If you have a good selection of colours, wonderful combinations can be arranged. It is almost like creating a painting; the finished article is really a statement by the creator. I work with one particular woman who is quite reserved. She, like most of the residents, has acute memory loss. But when it comes to putting colours together she always uses soft blues, purples and browns. Another woman uses completely contrasting combinations – bright reds, yellows and greens. The weavings really show their different temperaments and tastes.

Weaving techniques

To help with the weaving process, the warp threads can be alternated using two different colours of wool. The colours should be quite different, like red and yellow or blue and orange. These colours will not be seen on the completed work if the weft is beaten down properly. The weaver will get used to passing the shuttle under one colour as he or she weaves one way, and under the other colour on the return. Place a piece of white paper under the threads to prevent the warp thread from 'disappearing'. This will happen if the threads are similar in colour to the polystyrene tray or to the table-top.

The tension used when finishing a row is very important. Unfortunately, most of my participants confuse weaving with sewing, and instinctively pull the weft far too tight when finishing a row. This causes the selvage ends to pull in, or waist. If unchecked, the weaving will become narrower as each row is finished. Do make sure that the tension remains loose at the selvage ends.

When starting or finishing a weaving or changing weft colours, start and finish the weft a few warp threads in from the edge. Pass a short length of the yarn through to the back of the weaving. These yarn ends can be sewn in when the weaving is complete.

Shapes can be woven on the frame loom quite easily. They can be vertical, steep or shallow angles or even curved. An example of this is covered in the wall hanging project.

Each time a row of weaving is finished, the weft should be 'beaten' down to the preceding row to keep the threads tight against one another. This can be done with the fingers; and gives the weaver the chance to be directly in touch with the weaving, which I feel is very important.

Many of you will be aware of the simple loom using a flat card. This is usually introduced to young children at school. However, as I mentioned, I have found that a polystyrene meat tray, from a local supermarket, is preferable to flat card. It does not stand up to a lot of continued use, but it is readily available and ideal for small work. The construction of a larger, more permanent frame loom will be described later.

Weaving is often done by lifting up alternate warp threads with one hand and passing the weft wool through the shed that is formed with the other. Unfortunately, mature hands do get a little sore after a while, so I find a shuttle to be very helpful. A piece of heavy card is suitable for this; unfortunately, it does not stand up to a lot of heavy handling. For a sturdier shuttle I suggest making one from hardboard or Plexiglas.

Project 1
Constructing a simple loom

Constructing a tray loom and shuttle.

Materials required:
- Polystyrene meat tray
- Craft knife

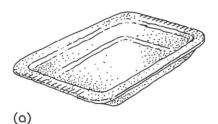

(a)

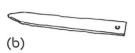

(b)

Figure 5.1

- Ruler
- Heavy card or hardboard
- Wool

For this project, the tray needs to be 265 mm × 150 mm wide (10$\frac{1}{2}$ in × 6 in). Refer to Figure 5.1a and cut slits or notches along both ends of the tray as shown. Determine the middle of the shortest width and measure outwards in either direction. The distance between the notches depends on how close you wish the warp threads to be. Obviously the closer together they are the more difficult it will be for the weaver to manipulate the shuttle through the threads. I would suggest a distance of 6 mm or 10 mm ($\frac{1}{4}$ in or $\frac{3}{8}$ in). The thickness of the yarn used for the warp threads will also have to be taken into account.

For the warp, use yarn that can withstand some tension, as the warp needs to be quite tight. Tie a warp thread to the tray, and pass it around the notch at the opposite end. Pass the yarn around the third notch and pull it taut. Continue warping the tray, missing every other notch. Keep the tension of the yarn as equal as possible throughout this process. Secure to the last notch. Now, using yarn of another colour, attach the warp threads to the remaining notches. If the yarn breaks tie another piece to it. Tie together at the notch ends of the tray. This will prevent knots from appearing in the weaving.

Make the shuttle about 150 mm (6 in) long by 20 mm ($\frac{3}{4}$ in) wide, or a little wider than the warp. A shuttle can be made from thick cardboard, or hardboard (see Figure 5.1b). The rough side of the hardboard should be sanded as smooth as possible. Do not use corrugated cardboard as it will deteriorate very quickly. Mount board used by a picture framer is a suitable material. Sand the edges smooth as any roughness will snag the warp threads.

Project 2
Weaving a small purse

Making a small purse.

Materials required:
- Several balls of wool
- Polystyrene weaving tray 190 mm × 270 mm ($7\frac{1}{2}$ in × $10\frac{1}{2}$ in)
- Shuttle
- Darning needle
- Snap fastener
- Sewing needle and thread

Procedure

The size of the purse, flat, unfolded is 60 mm × 100 mm ($2\frac{3}{8}$ in × $3\frac{7}{8}$ in). The weaving will be folded and sewn along the edge to make the purse, as shown.

Set up the warp threads to a width of 60 mm ($2\frac{3}{8}$ in). Insert a piece of cardboard through the warp threads. When the warp threads are untied or cut from the loom, the ends will then be of reasonable lengths so they can be sewn easily into the completed weaving.

Choose a colour scheme. If you are assisting people, allow them to give their opinion on the choice of colour. Cut a piece of yarn, and tie to the shuttle. Start the weaving process by passing the shuttle under one colour warp thread and over the next. Take care that the end warp threads (selvage) are not pulled in when finishing the row. Change to a different colour for the weft to create an interesting design. Continue weaving until the desired length of 100 mm ($3\frac{7}{8}$ in) is reached. Finish the weaving midway along the row, cut the yarn off the shuttle and pass the wool end through to the back of the weaving. Remove the warp threads from the tray, cutting at the notches.

Using the darning needle, sew the cut warp

threads into the weaving. Do the same for all of the loose yarn ends.

Lay the weaving on a flat surface with the front face uppermost. Fold the bottom edge of the weaving so that it is 30 mm ($1\frac{1}{4}$ in) from the top edge. Using the darning needle and wool, sew along the two sides. Turn the purse inside out, the front side of the weaving should now be on the outside. Using the needle and thread attach the fastener securely.

Project 3
Constructing a table loom

The following project, building a table loom, requires some woodworking tools and some basic woodworking skills. However, an alternative is to use a picture frame, or canvas stretcher bars.

Making a table loom.

Materials required:
- Canvas stretchers or a wooden picture frame 360 mm × 460 mm (approx. 14 in × 18 in) or four pieces of planed wood – two pieces 25 mm × 50 mm × 360 mm (1 in × 2 in × 14 in) and two pieces 25 mm × 50 mm × 460 mm (1 in × 2 in × 18 in)
- Panel pins 12 mm ($\frac{1}{2}$ in)
- Hammer
- Saw
- Ruler 8–12 mm ($\frac{1}{2}$ in) countersunk wood screws
- Wood glue
- Sandpaper
- Wool, two distinctly different colours

Procedure

If using the planed wood, join the pieces together with half joints as shown in Figure 5.2a. Glue and

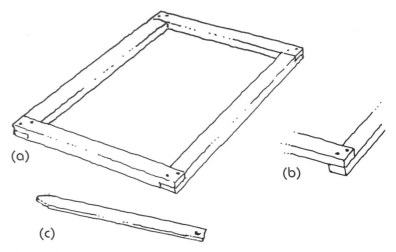

(a)

(b)

(c)

Figure 5.2

screw together. Allow the joints to dry overnight. Sandpaper to remove any rough edges. An alternative joining method is shown in Figure 5.2b.

When setting the nails for the distance between the warp threads, find the midpoints of the shortest sides of the frame. Measure out from these points distances of 6 mm or 10 mm ($\frac{1}{4}$ in or $\frac{3}{8}$ in). Hammer the nails in to about half of their length. Try to keep the height of each nail consistent. To prevent the wood from splitting the nails should be staggered.

The frame is now ready to tie the warp threads. As mentioned earlier, alternating the warp threads using two distinctly different colours will help the weaver enormously when threading the shuttle.

If you are preparing the loom for the next project (weaving a wall hanging) the full width of the frame should be used. Start by securely tying a thread of yarn at the first nail. Double the warp thread at this position as it will strengthen selvage ends. Wind the thread around the nail at the opposite end of the frame and return it to the first nail. Pull the warp thread tight and wind it around the nail. Miss the second nail and wrap the thread around the third nail, pulling it tight. Pass the thread around the third nail at the opposite end of the frame. Pull the thread tight and then wind it on to the fifth nail at

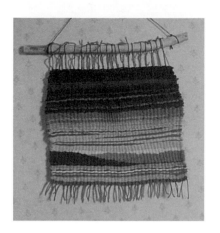

that end. Continue in this fashion until every second nail has a thread tied to it. Using the other colour, repeat the process until all the nails have a thread attached to them. Remember to double the warp thread at the other selvage end. To protect the weavers from catching their clothing or wrists on the nail heads, cover them with a piece of stout card. The frame is now ready for weaving. Make a shuttle from a piece of mount board or hardboard and shape it as indicated in Figure 5.2c.

Project 4
Wall hanging

Making a wall hanging.

Materials required:
- Table loom
- Shuttle
- Wool, several different colours
- Two A4 or one A3 sheet of paper
- Felt-tipped pens, assorted colours
- Thin card, the width of the frame

Procedure

I have suggested that the full width of the frame be used for this project. A narrower design could of course be woven if you wish. Decide on the size that the wall hanging is going to be and use a piece of paper the same size to design the wall hanging. Using the felt-tipped pens, draw a design onto the paper. Use colours that approximately match the colours of the wool available. I have suggested a lake and mountain scene. Create one of your own choosing if you wish, especially if your stock of coloured wools does not correspond to the design.

If the preceding project has been followed, the frame should be ready for weaving. Cut a piece of card about 60 mm ($2\frac{3}{8}$ in) wide to fit the full width of

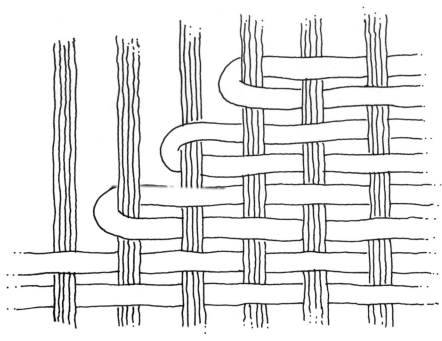

Figure 5.3

the warp threads. Insert this through the warp
threads. This will give you some warp ends when
the weaving is cut off the frame. They can either be
made into tassels, or sewn in to the weaving to make
a straight hem.

Lay the design behind the warp threads; this will
give the weaver a guide when choosing the weft
yarn. Tie a length of yarn to the shuttle and secure
the other end to the second or third warp thread in
from the edge. Leave a small length of this yarn
hanging on the wrong side of the work. This can
be sewn into the weaving later.

Referring to the design, begin weaving. If you are
using the lake and mountain scene, the green shoreline will be your first colour. Weave right across the
width of the warp until the incline in the design is
reached. Inclines of steep or shallow angles can be
made by varying the number of warp threads woven
(see Figure 5.3). The illustration shows a steep rise;
by weaving through fewer warp threads the angle
will be less steep. When this is complete the next

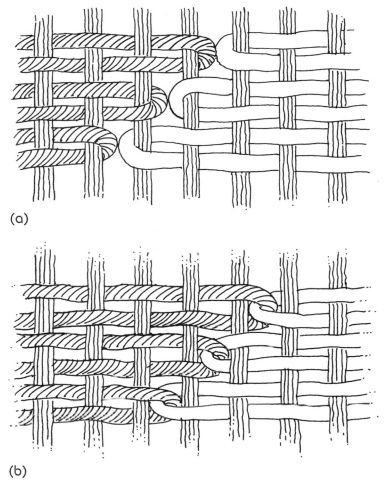

(a)

(b)

Figure 5.4

part of the design can be woven. Changing the weft to blue yarn, weave up to the start of the rise in the green foreground design.

There are now two possibilities to consider. The rows could be butted up to the green rows and then returned (see Figure 5.4a). This would leave a slit in the weaving which is quite acceptable. Another alternative is to interlock the different colours as shown in Figure 5.4b. This would mean untying the yarn from the shuttle and interlocking it with the same row of the butting weft.

Continue weaving this colour until the shoreline is reached. Change the yarn colour, and weave in the low mountain form. Use the same procedure as before for the incline. To give a feeling of distance as the mountain ranges recede, the principle of aerial perspective will be applied. This is covered in the tone study in chapter 2.

It is now a matter of comparing your yarn stock to get the lighter tone required. If this appears unworkable, do not worry too much. Use a light, cool colour that might indicate the form. Continue with the next mountain, and then fill in the sky around the mountains. The colour for the sky could be a single blue or a variety of blues. Both would work well. In the sample shown at the beginning of the project, yellow and red yarns have been used in the water and the sky, giving a feeling of a warm sunset.

Before removing the weaving, turn the loom over and darn in all the weft tails. The bottom warp threads could be made either into tassels by tying three or more together, or they could all be sewn in to make a straight edge.

If the weaving is to be hung, the top warp threads need to be tied to a dowel. If a more casual look is wanted, you might consider using a thin branch. Scrape off the bark and sandpaper smooth. Cut the branch longer than the width of the wall hanging. The branch or dowel may be either varnished or left in its natural condition. Attach a piece of yarn and the wall hanging is now ready to be hung.

Wall hanging designs can be as varied as you like, from the semi-realistic design just described to the very abstract. Weft material can also be just as varied; weaving in pieces of fabric, beads, wood, dried flowers, etc. can make a very interesting wall hanging.

Another simple project that the elderly enjoy is plaiting. Several different colours can be twined together and then plaited. They can be used as straps for woven bags or purses, coiled and sewn together to make coasters, or used to support wall hangings (see Figure 5.5).

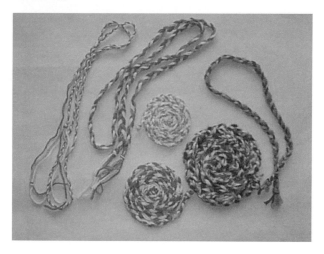

figure 5.5

Rug and tapestry making

I have memories of rug making with my parents when I was 10 years old. My father was convalescing from a TB operation, so I was introduced to a lot of craft work during his illness, and rug making was one of them. This particular rug process was hand tufted using a latch hook. It was my job to cut the wool, which of course had to be all the same length to ensure that the pile would be the same height. I recall winding the wool onto a stick which had a groove along one side. When it was full I was instructed to slit the wool with a razor using the groove as a guide. I thought, at the time, that it was great to have such an important job to do. After a period of time I was taught to use the latch hook and found it very satisfying to be able to help make something as important as a rug for the home. In looking back, I'm sure that there could not have been a great colour choice, as the rugs were basically made with just primary colour schemes plus brown. As the interest in rug making has grown again recently, there appears to be a good variety of colours from which to choose.

Another aspect of rug making is that the rugs make wonderful wall hangings. I have seen many rugs used in this way and they look fabulous. As they can be produced any size, the rug can be custom-made to fit a particular space whether it be a floor or a wall.

For a good hard-wearing rug 6-ply wool is used, with a canvas of 10 holes per 75 mm (3 in) where every hole is used. For lighter wear every other hole can be used. Canvas is available with more holes to the millimetre (inch) making the holes smaller, but it would then be difficult to get the rug hook through. The rug-making process can be done with the canvas on one's lap. It involves taking a piece of the cut wool and folding it in half; the rug hook is passed through the loop of the wool and into one of the canvas holes. The hook has a latch that opens as you push it into the hole. The hook is then pushed up through the next hole whereupon the two ends of the wool are placed in the open hook. The hook, together with the wool, is pulled through the canvas and back through the loop. This action automatically closes the latch, holding the two ends of wool securely in place, while the knot is formed. All that is now required is a slight pull on the wool to tighten the knot.

Rag rugs

Rag rugs are a very economical way of producing unique rugs. They can be made from recycled clothing or any fabric that does not fray too much. The process involves a canvas backing through which strips of fabric are pushed with a prodding instrument or pulled with a rug hook, a loop of material being formed to create the pile.

Any material to be considered for the rug should be washed beforehand. This is not only a matter of hygiene, but it will also rid the material of any moth eggs. The material should be pre-shrunk as much as possible. Any unwanted marks, tears or holes in the fabric can be cut away when the material is cut into strips. Once the fabric has been washed and dried it can be cut into strips.

Strips of fabric should be cut all the same width, as long and as possible, with similar materials. Try experimenting with cloth of different thickness as it will give a variety of effects. Try several widths before cutting up a lot of material.

Prodding method

The prodding technique is the simplest, but does not lend itself to intricate designs. It is a good idea to draw out a design on the hessian backing, before beginning. If you do not have a large quantity of material of the same colour, it may be better to have just a blend of the colours rather than a set design. As with all compositions, the completed rug should be balanced, so group the colours roughly in piles on the hessian. This will give you an idea of the completed design. Another possibility is to dye the material to colours of your choice; this would offer much more scope in creating a design of your liking. If a motif or design is to be used, it is best to do this first and fill in the surround later.

The rug can be worked on one's lap or on a frame. If a frame is used the hessian is secured by string or tacked with pins and the prodding is done from the 'wrong' side.

The procedure is simply to push the prodder through the hessian to make a hole; the material strip is then pushed through the hole. Another hole is made close to the first and the strip pushed through it. This process is continued until a row or area is finished or the strip is used. The height of the loop can be adjusted to one's own liking. It can be constant if used as a rug or a variety of different heights if used as a wall hanging; the latter would have a more sculptured and interesting look to the piece.

Punched needle method

A more modern method of rug making is to use a punch needle. This tool enables the height of the pile to be set by the depth that the needle passes through the backing, which can be any fabric. Hessian is suitable, as long as it is coarse enough so that the needle can be pushed through. Yarn is passed through the tube of the tool and pulled out through the eye opening at the other end. Working from the wrong side of the rug, the eye of the needle is positioned away from the direction of travel. The needle is held in an upright position and pushed through the backing material as far as it will go. The end of the yarn is held with one hand and the needle withdrawn so that it just clears the backing. Do not pull it any further than this or you will have too much yarn pulled through before reinserting the needle. Still holding the end of the wool, move the tool along a few threads and push the needle through the fabric once more. When the tool is inserted through the fabric as far as it will go, hold the loop that will be formed and pull out the needle. The weaving continues in this way until a change of colour is required or you need more wool. Remember that when you change direction, the needle will have to be turned, so that the eye is always facing away from the direction of travel.

Hooked method

In this method of rug making a rug hook is used. It is similar to a large crochet hook mounted in a wooden handle. Some rug weavers use hessian as a backing for hand-hooked rugs, but when working with older people I suggest that a canvas mesh is used. The mesh would have to be large enough to take the hook. Strips of material are cut as previously described. Hold a strip below the surface of the backing, push the hook through a hole; the material is caught and drawn back through the hole to form a loop. The height of the loop depends on one's own preference of pile height. If the rug is going to be a wall hanging, a variety of different heights would create an interesting and unique effect. Continue hooking until a change of colour is required or the strip has been woven. The end of the strip should be pulled through to the right side and cut to the same height as the rest of the pile.

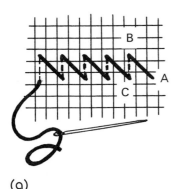

(a)

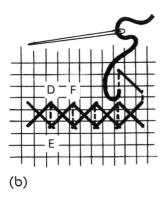

(b)

Figure 5.6

Tapestry rugs

For older people tapestry rug weaving is ideal. It is similar to needle point but has much larger stitches and is woven on a canvas mesh backing using rug or tapestry wool. The stitching is done with a tapestry needle using a basic tent or cross-stitch. Canvas backing can be selected depending on the amount of detail required – the finer the mesh the more intricate the detail can be.

As with all weaving projects, initial planning is essential. The size and shape should be decided upon, and the edges of the canvas turned under and stitched or taped to prevent fraying. I would suggest that a design be worked through on paper and coloured. This will assist greatly when working on the canvas, as the design can then be laid out accurately before starting the weaving. An interesting project would be to cut the canvas into 300-mm (12-in) squares, and have several people working on the pieces separately. The pieces could all be joined together when complete, to make a unique wall hanging or rug.

Figure 5.6 shows a typical cross-stitching procedure. Cut the wool into about 460-mm (18-in) lengths; do not break it as this will stretch the wool. Refer to Figure 5.6a. With the needle threaded, pass the needle up from the wrong side (A). Working from right to left, leave about 40 mm ($1\frac{1}{2}$ in) of wool at the back of the canvas. Insert the needle at (B) as indicated and then up through (C). Complete a row in this fashion and then reverse the direction and complete the cross as shown in Figure 5.6b. Insert at (D), up through (E) and down through (F). Change the colour of the wool as dictated by the design.

The tent stitch is another stitch that is frequently used for tapestry work. As the stitch uses every hole, it produces a hard-wearing finish, making it suitable for rugs as well as tapestries.

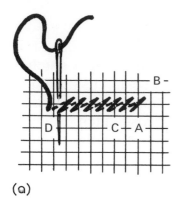

(a)

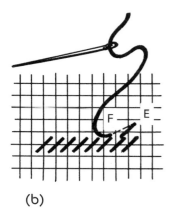

(b)

Figure 5.7

Referring to Figure 5.7, the stitch is worked from right to left again. The needle is passed up through (A). Leave a length of the wool at the back of the canvas and pass the needle down through a hole at (B). It is then brought up through (C). Continue in this fashion until the end of the row. At this point the needle is brought up through (D) (see Figure 5.7a). The canvas is now turned through 90 degrees. Passing the needle down through the mesh at (E) and up through (F) will start the tent stitch pattern again (see Figure 5.7b). Continue the stitch in this manner until a change of colour is desired.

When finishing a length of wool, sew the short ends through the wool threads at the back of the canvas. Cutting them off close to the canvas will keep the back of the rug tidy. Be careful not to pull or twist the wool as this will result in thin patches. Twisted wool can be unwound as you work by letting the needle spin out the twist naturally. If you do need to unpick an area, use a piece of new wool to replace it.

To finish the rug, back it with a lining material. The material should be cut larger than the rug. Turn the edges under and hem, mitring the corners. Attach the backing to the rug with a slip-stitch.

Hanging a rug

The preceding rug techniques will make attractive wall hangings. The hanging rail will depend on the weight of the rug. It is far better to use a rail that will take more weight than is actually required. Attach the rug with strong cord. Small weavings look very attractive attached to branches that have been pealed of their bark. The bare wood should be sanded. A clear varnish could be applied to complete the arrangement.

Card weaving

No doubt everyone has tried this method of weaving. It was certainly popular as a method of weaving raffia. However, because I like the feel of

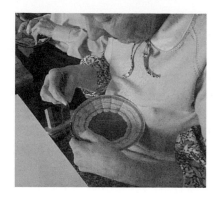

wool, and odd wool ends are so easy to come by, I decided to make my own cards for use with wool instead of raffia.

Materials required:
- Thick card (corrugated cardboard could be used, but extra care would have to be taken when weaving, as the cardboard tears easily)
- Pencil compass
- Pencil
- Craft knife
- Metal ruler
- Wool (preferably two or more colours)
- Bradawl or leather punch
- Darning needle
- Knitting needle

Procedure

Set the compass at 90 mm ($3\frac{1}{2}$ in) and describe a circle. Keeping the compass at the same centre point, describe a smaller circle with a 45 mm ($1\frac{3}{4}$ in) radius. Divide the circumference of the larger circle into seventeen equal parts – 30 mm ($1\frac{1}{4}$ in) is close. Adjust as necessary. Whatever spacing is decided upon, there must be an odd number of points. From each of these points draw a line towards the centre of the circles, stopping at the smaller circle's circumference. Cut around the circumference of the large circle. Using the craft knife and metal ruler cut twice along the radiating lines to make slots. These are to take the thickness of the wool. Make sure that the slot is cut precisely to the edge of the inner circle where the weaving will begin.

The centre circle of card can be painted or decorated with decoupage. Follow the instructions for decoupage in chapter 3. Wait until the centre is totally dry before proceeding.

Insert a piece of wool through one of the slots at the inner circle, leaving an end of about 30 mm

$(1\frac{1}{4}$ in) on the underside. Start the weaving process. When you have come full circle, continue on to the next row. Because there are an odd number of slots, the weave will automatically go over the card that you went under on the first round. Be sure to pull the wool firmly down so that each row is tight against the previous row. A knitting needle is handy for this job, as hands get a little sore after a while. The tail end of wool that you left on the underside can be woven in as you go or sewn in later. When a few rows have been completed, consider changing the colour of the wool. Each segment should be covered with an equal number of rows before changing colours, and one should also be level with the starting point of that colour. While weaving, try to shape the outer edge of the card upwards to form a shallow dish.

Continue weaving until the card is almost full then cut the wool and sew all the ends through to the underside of the weaving. The rim can now be finished with a blanket stitch. To aid in sewing, holes can made with the bradawl close to the top of last row. If the finishing colour has been decided upon, the card edge can be painted to match it before weaving the last row.

Chapter 6

Stencilling and block printing

Stencilling
Silk screen printing
Stamping and printing

Stencilling

Stencilling is one of the easiest forms of decoration as it requires very little artistic skill. I have used stencilling very successfully in my own activities programme. As most of the residents have difficulty copying or drawing a design, I find the use of stencils very convenient, especially if the design is going to be repeated several times. The design can be painted either through the stencil, using a special stencilling brush, or the contour can be pencilled onto the surface and painted afterwards. If you use the latter technique, the stencil should be made of thick card or plastic, as thinner material is difficult to trace around.

You can buy pre-cut stencils, or you can cut them yourself. When purchasing pre-cut stencils be aware that the thickness of the stencil will govern the result. If they are too thick, smudging will result, as pigment is likely to build up around the edge of the cut-out. If the stencil is too thin it will become floppy especially at the 'bridges', the connecting links between the cut-outs.

If you are cutting your own stencil, it is preferable to use Mylar. This material is transparent and flexible and resists tearing. It takes spray adhesive well. The stencil can be attached temporarily to the surface with masking tape or spray glue and then removed after the paint application. It is ideal for stencilling on curved surfaces.

Stencils cut from card are workable but they have the disadvantage that the working surface cannot be seen. If producing a design with more than one colour, registration marks have to be made. When cutting stencils use a very sharp craft knife. Straight lines are best cut with the aid of a steel ruler. For intricate shapes use a scalpel knife with a fine blade.

When cutting curved lines, turn the stencil instead of the blade. A cutting board should be used at all times; this could be a piece of glass, heavy cardboard or the special cutting surface available at art shops. This material can be used many times as the surface tends to close after a cut is made. If using glass the knife will have to be sharpened frequently.

Paper doilies also make interesting stencils. They can be used whole or cut into small sections to suit the application. The doily will eventually break down with continuous applications of paint. To improve its durability apply several coats of clear varnish to both sides, letting the doily dry between applications. You could also try making your own paper stencil from cartridge paper.

There are several types of paint that work well with stencilling, but as with the other projects in this book I have purposely stayed away from solvent-based pigments. Instead, I suggest that you use water-based colours. This makes cleaning up much easier and avoids toxic fumes.

I recommend using acrylic paints. The paint dries very quickly, is very opaque and dries to a plastic-like waterproof coating. An advantage of this medium is that it dries almost as fast as one can work, smudging is minimised and one colour can be applied over the top of another without their mixing. Also, as the paint is so opaque, it can be used on coloured surfaces. Please note that there are specially formulated acrylics for different applications. Do make sure that the pigments you purchase are suitable for the material you are working on.

An important consideration for stencil work is the type of brush that is used. The bristles need to be quite long and not too soft. When applying paint, the brush can then be used with a good deal of pressure for darker shades and very lightly to give lighter tones. Specially designed brushes are available from your local art shop or speciality shop.

Paint can also be applied with a natural sponge. Holes in the sponge give a very interesting texture when applying paint. The sponge can also be used to give the material an overall colour. When using the sponge, load it with a minimal amount of paint, as directed when using the brush.

As some older people may not be able to draw intricate shapes or manipulate a sharp knife, they may well need some help with the following project. If this is the case, I feel that it is important that they watch the process develop and perhaps select or suggest a design to use.

Project 1
Making a paper stencil

Materials required:
- Copier paper
- Scissors
- Craft knife
- Pencil, 2B
- Ruler
- Clear varnish, water-based
- Brush, household

Procedure

Cut a 200 mm (8 in) square from the paper, fold it in half and then in half again. You should now have a smaller square of folded paper. Fold the square diagonally. Cut curved or straight shapes out of the folded diagonal edge. Vary the size and distance apart. Open the diagonal fold so that you can now work on the small square. Cut more shapes out of the edges that are folded. When the paper is unfolded you will have a symmetrical design cut out of the

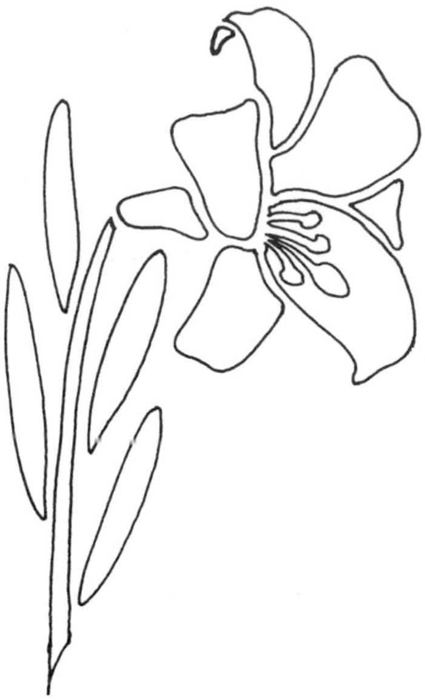

Figure 6.1

paper. Apply several coats of varnish, letting each application dry before applying another.

Project 2
Making a stencil from a photograph

Making a stencil from a photographic image (Figure 6.1).

Materials required:
- Mylar, heavy plastic or stencil card
- Sharp craft knife
- Steel ruler
- Tracing paper
- HB pencil
- Cutting board

Procedure

In chapter 2, I describe how to create a line drawing from a photograph. This changes the photograph into flat graphic form. From this, the individual elements can be divided by the lines. Try this with the lily: draw the lily larger, tracing each segment of the form. As you complete a segment, move the tracing paper, so that a small gap appears between the traced segment and the lily form of the original. Trace the next segment with the tracing paper thus offset. Do this with the rest of the shapes. You should now have the complete design made up of segments with spaces between them. Transfer the traced design to the stencil card or Mylar. The resulting image can be used as a positive or negative. In other words, after the lily is cut out to form the stencil and paint is brushed on through the stencil, colour will appear on the petals and leaves. Alternatively, the shape around the lily could be cut out. Paint would then appear as the background, leaving the lily the colour of the material. The stencil would have to have a border; bridges would have to be cut to attach the parts of the flower together and to the border. If you feel courageous enough hair could be used for the bridges (see section on silk-screen printing).

This technique can be applied to many motifs that might interest you. Leaf patterns from Greek and Roman columns and friezes can be explored, as well as designs from the Art Nouveau period. A good source of reference material can usually be found at your local library.

Project 3
Making a greeting card

Stencil printing a greeting card.

Materials required:
- Stencil, a design of your choice
- Stencil brush
- Acrylic paint
- Spray adhesive
- Masking tape
- Card stock, A4 size
- Ruler
- HB pencil
- A medium size cardboard box
- Paper towel
- Saucers
- Dinner knife

Procedure

Tape the card lengthways to a flat surface, measure halfway and lightly draw a line to divide the card in half. The right half will be the front of the card where the stencil will be attached. Spray the reverse side of the stencil with spray adhesive. Use the cardboard box on its side as a mini spray booth. The stencil can be attached to a piece of cardboard with a bulldog clip or paper clip. This can then be placed inside the box for spraying. If you do not wish to use spray adhesive, the stencil may be secured in place with masking tape.

Fold a piece of paper towel, and put it within reach; placing it in a saucer is helpful. Decide on the colour to be used. If the pigment is in jars, the brush may be used directly, picking up a small amount of the colour. If it is a tube, squeeze a small amount onto a saucer, and pick up a small amount with the brush. Work the loaded brush on the paper towel; this will have the effect of spreading the pigment through the bristles and removing any excess paint. The biggest problem with stencilling is the use of too much paint, whereupon the paint will bleed under the stencil. When applying the paint, use the brush held vertically. There are basically two strokes one can use − a short dabbing action, which will give mottled effect, or a circular movement. The latter gives a smooth finish. Try them both as the effects are quite different. Remember not to overload the brush. Dry it first on the paper towel before applying more paint. From time to time check to see how the design is transferring by lifting up one end of the stencil. Clean the stencil if paint is building up on the edges, as this will lead to smudging. When you feel that you have applied enough paint, remove the stencil carefully. Clean it thoroughly.

Wait until the paint has dried thoroughly. To make a neat fold in thick card, score the card along the pencil line, using the blunt side of a dinner knife against a ruler. Do not press too hard. The fold can now be made evenly from the back of the card. To make the fold sharper, lay a piece of clean paper on the back of the folded card. With a little pressure and the knife almost flat, run it over the folded edge. Erase the pencil line and any marks as necessary.

Once you have mastered the basics of stencilling, you can go on to try a variety of stencil projects. There are many applications for stencil work, such as adding a design to a plain wooden tray; applying decoration to place mats, small boxes, or terracotta pots; making wrapping paper; adding designs to greeting cards; borders on photograph mounts and tiles. There are many possibilities where stencils can also be used with fabric. Designs can be applied to pillowcases, tablecloths, cushion covers and lampshades. Do remember to check that the paint used is suitable for the application. You will also need to know how to fix the paint. Some pigments require steam fixing, others can be heat-fixed with an iron.

Silk-screen printing

Silk-screen printing is, in fact, a refined stencil printing process. It is based on the Japanese stencilling technique dating back hundreds of years. Intricate shapes were cut and the delicate pieces were held together with human hair or silk. The printing ink was not impeded by the fine hairs, so the design would be free of any 'bridges' that occur with regular stencils. It was not developed in the West until the beginning of the twentieth century. The textile industry soon adopted it as a method of printing on fabric. Other industries also saw its commercial possibilities and began to use the process widely.

Artists now use it for short limited edition prints. As an art printing process it is called serigraphy to distinguish it from the commercial process. Light-sensitive emulsion in applied to the screen and a photographic image of the artwork is exposed onto the emulsion. Intricate detail can be obtained in this manner, as well as close registration multicolour images.

Although this method of printing has become very commercialised, and the equipment quite specialized, it is a printing process that is quite simple. One can start a simple printing programme without a lot of equipment or at great expense.

All that is needed is a printing screen frame to which a stencil has been adhered, a 'squeegee' and printing ink. An amount of ink is poured into the frame and the material to be printed is placed under the frame. Ink is then pulled across the screen, which is now in contact with the material, by the squeegee. The ink is squeezed through the screen onto the material; the shape of the image transferred being defined by the stencil. The printed result will depend on the mesh of the screen: a coarse screen will give edges that are stepped whereas a fine screen will give clean edges. The latter, however, can be hard to push ink through and does tend to get clogged with ink. A balance has to be achieved between the printing quality and the skill of those doing the actual printing.

Printing inks are available with either a water or a spirit base. As with other projects in this book, I recommend that water-based materials are used. This will minimise the use of toxic substances. There are specially formulated inks for different applications, so do ensure you have the correct ink for your project. Inks are transparent or opaque. Transparent inks will not cover dark colours, they will also change colour optically; that is, if you were to print yellow on a blue material, it would appear green when printed. Opaque inks cover coloured material very well, so you could print light-coloured ink on a dark material.

Printing frames can be purchased complete with a mesh for a specific application. If cared for properly the mesh will last for many projects. Do remember to clean the mesh thoroughly after a project, making sure that ink is removed from every square of the mesh by running water at the highest pressure through it. Ink should not be allowed to dry in the mesh, as it would be extremely difficult to remove. A special ink retarder when mixed with the ink will slow the drying process in the screen. If the ink does start to dry, making printing difficult, it is best to remove the ink from the frame and clean the screen thoroughly. Dry the screen – a hairdryer will speed things up and restart the printing process.

The frame can be used either on a table or taken to any other surface to be printed. As this book is intended for older people, I recommend that projects be chosen so that printing is done on a table. For multiple printing it is more convenient if the frame is attached to a base or the table with a removable pin hinge. The frame can then be removed from the printing base for cleaning. Attaching a swivel support leg to the outside of the frame will enable it to be propped up between printings, leaving both hands free to remove a print and place another piece of material in position.

Project 4
Printing a greeting card

Printing a greeting card by silk-screening.

Materials required:
- Printing frame
- Two hinges with removable pins
- Squeegee
- Printing ink
- Masking tape
- Paper, for stencil
- Varnish
- Household brush
- Heavy card, A4 size
- Pencil, 2B
- Craft knife
- Ruler
- Newspaper

Procedure

As more than one print is to be produced, it is a good idea to prepare the frame for registration. Locate and mark the centre of each side on its outside edge. When these lines are joined it will give you the centre of the frame. Attach the hinges to the top of the frame and to the table or base. Transfer the centre marks from the frame to the printing table and connect these four marks. Remove the hinge pins.

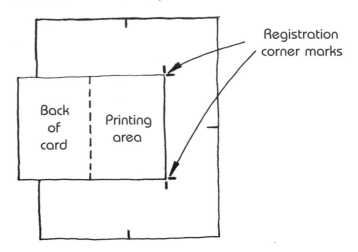

Registration
corner marks

Back
of
card

Printing
area

Figure 6.2

Registration marks for placement of the card now have to be made on the printing table. Take a piece of the A4 card and make a light pencil mark at the exact centre of the two shortest edges. As the card is to be folded in half, the image needs to be printed in the centre of the right-hand half of the card. Place a mark on the longest edge at one quarter of the total length in from the right-hand edge. This mark will be the centre of the folded card. Lay the card on the table, aligning the marks of the card with those on the table. Now make a registration mark on the frame base or board (see Figure 6.2). To prepare the screen for printing, tape along the top inside edges of the frame in such a way that half the width of the tape sticks to the frame and the other half to the screen. This will prevent ink from seeping through at the edges. Choose a design from the pattern section of the book and re-size it to fit on half of the A4 card. Prepare the stencil as in project 1 of this chapter. Attach it with tape to the underside of the frame, centring it by using the registration marks that you put on the frame. On the inside of the frame, mask off the rest of the screen, overlapping the tape to prevent any seepage. As the printing is done when the squeegee is pulled towards you, the masking tape should be overlapped so that the action of the squeegee does not lift the tape.

Attach the frame to the printing base by reinserting the hinge pins. It is always advisable to pull a proof print before printing on the actual material, it will also fill the screen with ink for the first real print. A proof can be done on scrap paper, so place a sheet under the frame in readiness for this. With the frame flat on the printing surface, place the squeegee in position at the top of the frame, i.e., furthest away from you. Spoon or squeeze some ink in front of the squeegee, the length of which should be a little more than the width of the design to be printed. Pull the squeegee towards you, pushing down firmly on the screen with a uniform pressure. Do not stop pulling until the squeegee is well past the design. Lift the squeegee with the residue of the ink, and place it back at the top of the frame. Lift the frame and check the printed image. If areas of the design are missing or the image is weak, repeat the printing process. Always ensure that there is more than enough ink in the screen before starting to print. When you are happy with the resulting print, place a piece of the card stock on the printing table. Make sure that the card butts up to the registration corners and print the image. Lie the cards on a clean, flat surface to dry or hang up on a line with clothes pegs.

Cleanse the screen of all ink, and remove the masking tape, leave to dry.

Stamping and block printing

Material required:

- Water-based paint
- Brushes
- Printing roller
- Sheet of glass
- Craft knife
- PVA glue
- Dinner or palette knife
- Vegetables: potato, carrot, parsnip, mushroom, pepper

Activities for Older People

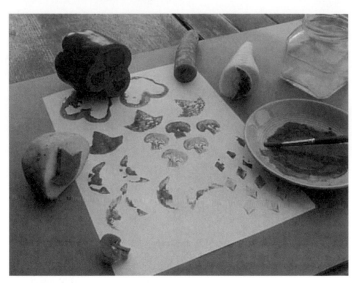

Figure 6.3

Stamps can be purchased or made from a variety of materials, including vegetables. I have used stamping and block printing as well as stencilling very successfully with older people. They like being able to use a stamp to create a design of their own. Small simple stamp designs are best, especially if people are new to this type of printing. I have shown what can be done with a variety of vegetables (see Figure 6.3). Some have been used without any cutting – mushrooms, cauliflower florets and peppers. They have been simply cut to give a flat surface suitable for printing. You can use a variety of paints. Mix the paint to a creamy consistency and do not apply too much at one time. Paint can be applied with a brush or the stamp can be dipped into the paint. Depending on the type of paint used, you will be able to use the vegetable stamp to apply a design to many different surfaces. There are many other natural stamps that can be used without even having to create a design. Try leaves, grasses, flowers, feathers, a piece of hessian or netting. Anything that has a textured surface will do. You will need lots of newspaper to protect working surfaces. I would also suggest that aprons are worn by the participants.

I have also seen interesting designs created with string. A piece of string is shaped into a design and attached to a block of wood with PVA glue, or if a larger design is required a piece of board can be used. Once it is dry, paint is applied with the roller as described earlier.

Cut a potato with a large knife to get a flat cut surface. Place it, cut surface down, onto a piece of paper and transfer the outline by drawing with a pencil around it. This will give you the shape and area for a design. A design can now be tried out on the paper before cutting into the vegetable. Keep it simple, as it is difficult to get intricate shapes with vegetables. If the design is not symmetrical or if you want letters and words, they will have to be cut in reverse in order to print the right way round.

Stamps made from vegetables and organic matter will obviously deteriorate quickly. If you want to reuse a stamp design over a period of time, you may like to make or purchase a rubber stamp.

Rubber stamps

There now seems to be a resurgence of the rubber stamp printing industry, as dozens of ready-made stamps are now available from art and speciality shops. In my youth I remember being ecstatic about getting a 'John Bull' printing outfit one Christmas – I believe they are still available today. For many hours I toiled with tweezers, assembling tiny letters in a wooden printing block. Unfortunately the finished result would often be nondescript words and sentences, as I would often run out of the necessary letters. I must say, though, I got pretty good at reading in reverse.

If you would like to make your own design, rubber stamp material is available. It is easy to cut and clean designs can be produced from it. The self-adhesive backing makes it easy to stick to a block for ease of printing.

Printing with cardboard

Small simple designs can be printed using corrugated cardboard. Draw or trace the design onto a piece of cardboard. Cut the design with a sharp craft knife, and glue it to a block of wood. An abstract design using several shapes could also be created. Paint can then be rolled on, as described earlier. Different colours may also be applied to the various shapes to make the printed design more interesting. Unfortunately, this material has only a limited printing life, as the cardboard will break down with repeated applications of paint.

Lino block printing

Lino printing has been used for many years. Lino especially made for printing can be purchased from art suppliers. The lino is glued to a wooden block and a printing image formed by gouging out the lino with special carving tools. The design is usually drawn out on paper and then transferred to the lino using carbon or transfer paper. Lino cuts more easily when warmed a little; this can be done with a hairdryer.

If lino cutting is new to you, I would suggest practising on a scrap piece of lino first. The various lino tools available offer the opportunity to explore different cuts. The smaller V-shaped tool can be used for intricate shapes, while the broader shape can be used for removing large areas.

Unless you have a lot of experience with this material, a design for a lino block should be quite simple. The following project is printing up a greeting card using the Art Nouveau design from the pattern section at the end of the book.

For short print runs, say 20 or 30, a dessert spoon can be used quite successfully to burnish the image from the block.

Project 5
Making a lino block

Making a lino block and printing an image.

Materials required:
- Lino
- Plywood
- Lino gouges
- Ink roller
- Pencil, 2B, 2H
- Red colouring pencil
- Tracing or transfer paper
- Glass sheet about A4 size
- Block printing ink, blue
- Thin white card, A5 size
- Dessert spoon
- PVA glue
- Household brush

Procedure

Cut a piece of thick plywood 105 mm × 150 mm (4 $\frac{1}{8}$ in × 5$\frac{7}{8}$ in), i.e., the same dimensions as the folded card. Make sure that the corners are square, as you will be lining up the edges of the card with the block before burnishing. Cut the lino 85 mm × 130 mm (3$\frac{5}{8}$ in × 5 in) and glue it to the plywood, centring it so that there is an equal border. Apply some weight (books will do) to bond the lino to the block.

Clean the surface of the lino with methylated spirits or soapy water. Transfer the Art Noveau design from the pattern section of the book onto the tracing or transfer paper. Adjust and simplify it where necessary. Turn the tracing paper over, image side onto the lino, and draw over the lines with a 2H pencil.

Carefully cut out the design with a lino-cutting tool, removing the part that you do not wish to print. Working away from the body will help prevent the risk of injury. Clamps can be purchased to hold the block, or a stop can be constructed as

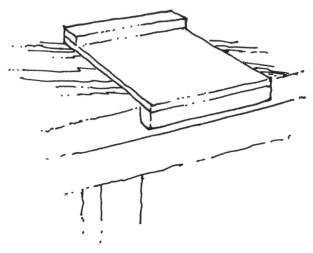

Figure 6.4

shown (see Figure 6.4). This would leave both hands free, making for safer carving. When you have completed the cutting, the lino can be inked up.

Mix the colours on a sheet of glass. This should be done before inking up the printing block. To do so, put a small amount of paint onto a clean sheet of glass, fold the paint a little with the knife. If you are mixing two or more colours together, blend them well, folding the colours together with the knife. Work the paint with the roller until a thin coat of paint covers the glass. Continue rolling in different directions until the roller is evenly coated. Roll up the printing block, making sure that the image is completely coated with ink.

Centre the card over the block. Place another piece of card on top of this. The fold should be on the right side with the image right side up.

Once the paper is in position, do not move it, as the ink would smudge. Take the spoon in one hand, gripping it firmly. With the thumb in the hollow, burnish over the card with the back of the spoon. Pressure may have to be exerted if printing on thick card; experiment first to get the right impression.

Lay out the printed cards individually to dry. When they are completely dry, fold from the back of the card.

Mono printing

Mono printing is often used by artists to create short-run reproductions of their work. Paint a design onto a piece of glass or plastic film. Before the paint has time to dry, lay the material you wish the design to be transferred to onto the wet paint. Apply light pressure to transfer the image. The second print will be much lighter than the first, so no two prints are identical. Abstract designs work very well for this type of printing. Paint is spread on the glass using a comb made from cardboard or you can purchase one from your art suppliers. You could also make designs and textures with such things as a pencil, twig or a natural sponge. Small objects such as leaves or cut paper shapes could be applied before the print is taken. Work quickly, as the paint may dry before you have a chance to take the print.

Picture transfer

Materials required:

- Transfer medium
- Household brush, small
- Household sponge
- A printed image

This is not really a printing process, but rather a method of transferring a printed picture to another surface.

Apply a coat of the transfer medium to the front of the picture, leave to dry for between 15 and 20 minutes. Apply another coat of medium, brushing in an opposite direction from the first. Leave to dry. Repeat the process two or three times. Leave to dry for 24 hours. Trim the varnished picture leaving about 5 mm ($\frac{1}{4}$ in) around the edge. Immerse the paper in warm water for about 20 minutes. This will facilitate removal of the paper. Using you finger or sponge remove the paper from the back of the photograph. Leave to dry for about 4 hours.

To apply the transfer to the surface, brush on a coat of the medium to the back of the transfer. Position it in place and remove any air bubbles with a hard roller. A wallpaper seam roller works very well. Leave it to dry for 24 hours. To protect the transfer, apply several coats of clear varnish. Leave each coat to dry before applying the next.

Peel-off stickers

If you require something simpler than the above ideas, then peel-off stickers may help. A large selection is available from the art suppliers listed at the back of the book. These are ideal for making greeting cards, pictures or bookmarkers, and are very easy to use. Stickers are self adhesive and available as motifs, words or borders. They are obtainable in gold, silver, rainbow or plain colours. Three-dimensional decoupage stickers are also available. It is simply a matter of peeling off the design from the backing and applying it to the surface.

As large selections of greeting-card blanks and envelopes are available, the end product is very professional and ideal for fund-raising items.

Chapter 7

Glass and silk painting

Glass painting
Materials, preparation and painting
Silk painting

Glass painting

This type of craft work looks very complex at first sight, and many people are put off trying it because of its professional-looking quality. I use this type of painting in my activities programme and have had very good results. The fear of attempting such work seems to diminish when I explain that I will be doing the design and layout work, and all the person has to do is to put in the colour.

The concept is, of course, a simplified form of stained glass work that can be found in churches and historical buildings. Instead of cutting coloured glass and fitting it into lead moulding, a special paint, which dries to a plastic-like finish, is used.

The paint is available either as water-based or solvent-based and in several colours; they each mix well with one another. The solvent-based paint dries

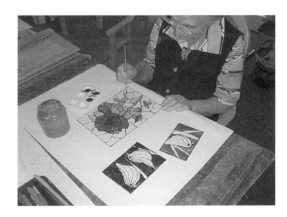

in 8 hours and the water-based in an hour; the paint is tack-free in 20 minutes. The solvent-based stained glass paint offers a better resistance to a light washing in cold water. I have washed water-based paint in cold water with no adverse effect. The manufacturer states that neither product should be considered for a utilitarian object. A matt varnish is available which gives a frosted glass effect.

To replicate the stained glass effect, a design is drawn and the glass, or Plexiglas, is placed over the design. Cerne relicf, a semi-liquid plastic available in tubes, is then used to outline the design. This, when dry, becomes hard and looks very much like stained glass leading. Glass paint is then applied to the segments divided by the outliner. This paint can then be allowed to dry, or another colour can be added while it is still wet. Mixing colours like this gives dramatic and unusual results. When the design has been finished and the paint is completely dry, it could be placed in a window. A hole can be drilled in it and the piece hung on a thread or suction cup hook. A small pane could also be replaced in a door or window. When sunlit, it will cast a rainbow of colours throughout the room. These suncatchers add a wonderful ambience to a room and are, naturally, very saleable items for fund-raising events.

There are many other applications for glass painting including decorating empty wine bottles and making decorative boxes. Both these applications will be covered in the following projects. But first, a word about the preparation and painting procedure.

Materials, preparation and painting

The items one uses for glass painting can be quite varied. As long as the surface is grease free, the paint will adhere to non-porous and some porous materials. However, transparent material will allow the paint to be seen at its best, especially when lit from the back. Thin plastic can be used; it is inexpensive, but it will need to be supported, as it will

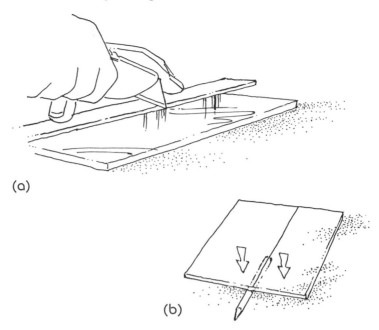

(a)

(b)

Figure 7.1

curl. Off-cuts of 2 mm ($\frac{1}{16}$ in) glass from your local picture framing shop or glass shop, are usually available at a minimal cost. They might even be happy for you to take them away. Plexiglas off-cuts are often available from the same source as glass, but there will probably be a small charge. Plexiglas is preferable when making suncatchers. If a suction hook is used for a window display be aware that it can come loose and fall. Predrilled glass suncatcher blanks and glass boxes are usually available from your art suppliers. I have found empty plastic chocolate boxes to be quite acceptable and readily available, especially after Christmas and Valentine's day.

For suncatchers, I recommend you use 2-mm Plexiglas. It is easily cut by scoring it a few times with a craft knife (Figure 7.1a). Make sure that the knife cuts right to the edge of the Plexiglas, at the start and finish of the scored line. Place a piece of heavy card or hardboard under the Plexiglas to protect the working surface. Use a steel ruler and work on a firm flat surface. Measure accurately, marking with a fine felt-tipped pen. Lay a pencil underneath and along the scored line and press firmly on either side of the line (see Figure 7.1b). If breaking a long piece of Plexiglas, you might have to move the pencil along and repeat the process. It should snap easily. The edges will be a little rough, so smooth them with emery paper.

When choosing or creating a design, keep the shapes and lines simple and avoid lots of detail. By simplifying the design, the finished product will be much stronger. Before a design is started, the size and shape of the piece has to be considered. When this has been cut, place it on a piece of paper and draw around the shape with a pencil. This will give you the space in which your design has to fit. Complete the design. Any changes should be done at this time. When the design is finalised, place the glass back on the paper and secure with masking tape.

In the following project, making a suncatcher, the complete process will be described.

Cerne relief outliner should be used on grease-free surfaces, so clean the glass thoroughly before starting the application. Outliner is available in tubes of three colours: black, gold or silver. It is also available as a glass leading replica. When choosing the outline colour, be aware that gold and silver cerne relief will show any over-painting. When painting the various segments care has to be taken to prevent paint getting onto the relief outline. If working on a suncatcher with gold or silver outliner, and paint does get on the outliner, hang the suncatcher with the relief outline to the window. Then the mistakes will not be seen. The outliner is quite fluid when squeezed from the tube and dries hard in an hour or so, depending on the thickness of the line. The line thickness is governed by how much of the tip is cut off the plastic nozzle. Applying the outliner takes a little practice, so cut a small amount off the tip of the nozzle at an angle. The line will then be quite fine. Keep a paper towel close by as the nozzle will need to be cleaned from time to time. Apply the liner to the glass and squeeze the tube from the end. Keeping a light, even pressure, move the tube slowly along your design lines. Keep the tube moving and the line flowing to avoid a build up or a missed space anywhere. If you wish to change or correct a line wait until the outliner is dry. It can be lifted off with a blunt knife and the line corrected. When the design is complete, remove the tape. Outliner should now be applied to the edges of the glass.

Wait until the outliner is totally dry before applying the glass paint.

The pigment, when applied to a non-porous surface such as glass, requires a different brush stroke from a regular painting project. I recommend that a small amount of paint is poured into a palette and then applied from there. The paint should be applied with a small round brush with a light dabbing action, with the brush fully loaded. If the paint is brushed too much, the result will be streaky. The consistency of the paint has to be just right; if it is too thin it will flow too quickly and leave bare patches, or if it is too thick it will not flow at all. It should spread within the segment with a minimal amount of brush work.

Check on a scrap piece of glass before starting a project. Some colours require more thinning than others: they are easily thinned by adding a few drops of water and stirring well.

Continue adding paint, letting it settle to the edges of the outline; care should be taken to cover the surface right up to the outline. Complete one segment at a time adding more paint until it is completely covered. The paint will start to dry as soon as it is exposed to the air, so any additional paint should be added without delay. While applying the paint, keep the glass flat; do not pick it up until the paint is completely dry.

If the result is not to your liking, wait until the paint is completely dry. The intensity of a colour can be increased by adding another layer of the same colour on top of the first. Or, as the paint is transparent, another colour painted on top of the first will change the colour totally.

If the piece is not improved by any of these actions, use a knife to separate a portion of paint from the glass. Peel the paint film off and repaint. Plexiglas will be scratched by a metal object so use a plastic knife to lift the paint. A fresh application of paint will help hide scratches and blemishes.

Glass paint can be mixed 'wet-in-wet', with wonderful results, if the right colour combinations are used. Larger areas are better for this. Experiment on a spare piece of glass to blend colours to your liking.

As I recommend using water-based paints, brushes can be cleaned in water. They should be cleaned frequently, especially when working on a large piece. The paint will start to dry in the brush, making paint application difficult. When a project is completed, the brushes should be cleaned in warm soapy water and dried.

Try to keep the lip of the pot of glass paint clean. If this is not done on a regular basis difficulty will be experienced in removing the cap. If this happens run the pot under the hot water tap. The lid can usually be unscrewed after a short while.

Project 1
Poppy suncatcher

Making a poppy suncatcher.

Materials required:
- Plexiglas or glass blank
- Glass paint: deep blue, night blue, orange, emerald green. Water-based paints are assumed
- Palette
- Brush – No 4 round short-handled craft brush
- Water pot
- Craft knife
- Metal ruler
- Cutting board
- Paper, or tracing A4 size
- HB pencil
- Sandpaper

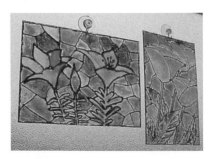

Procedure

From the pattern section, copy or trace the poppy design onto a piece of paper. If you are using a ready-cut glass blank, the design may have to be adjusted to fit the proportions of the glass blank.

Measure and cut the Plexiglas: 75 mm × 100 mm (3 in × 4 in) Remove any protective paper and sand the edges smooth. Clean with soap and warm water to remove any grease. Dry and lay the glass over the design and tape together securely.

The outliner can now be applied. As explained earlier, the application of the outliner can be a little difficult to control. Do not worry if the line is not absolutely perfect. Irregular lines will not be noticed too much once the painting is complete.

Check to see if the paint is of the right consistency, and pour a little of each blue into the palette. Starting with one of the blues, fill in the background of each alternate segment. Check that each segment is completely covered up to the outline as corners can be easily missed. Also check for small bubbles and any areas that might require additional paint. When you are satisfied with the paint application, put the piece aside to dry for 20 minutes or so.

Continue painting the background using the other blue. When completed, lay the glass aside for it to dry a little. Check the consistency of the orange paint and pour a little into the palette. Apply the orange paint to the poppy segment and make sure that the intensity is strong; apply more paint until this is achieved. Finish the poppy design by painting in the leaf and stem. Lay the suncatcher aside to dry overnight.

The Plexiglas will need a hole drilled in it if you are going to hang it in a window. It can be hung by a thread on a suction hook. If a suction cup hook is used, check the diameter and use the correct drill size. To drill the hole, apply a piece of masking tape, where the hole is to be drilled, to the reverse side of the glass suncatcher. If the tape is applied to the painted side there is a possibility that it will lift off the paint when it is removed. Measure accurately, and find the centre of the glass across the top edge. This will ensure that the suncatcher will hang vertically. Measure from the top edge down about 5 mm ($\frac{3}{16}$ in) on the centre line. Place a piece of wood under the drilling point, get an assistant to hold it steady and drill through. The suncatcher can now be hung in a window.

Try different shapes, such as diamond, square or oval suncatchers. To add another aspect to your design, Plexiglas can be filed into any shape that you choose.

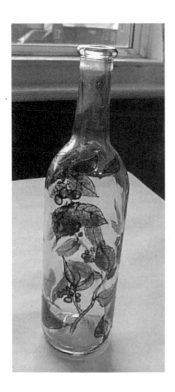

Project 2
Autumn leaf wine bottle

Wine bottles, and any other bottles, can be delightfully transformed with the application of glass paint. The following project will show you how to do just that.

Materials required:
- A used clear glass wine bottle, or any clear glass bottle.
- Glass paint – reddish brown, orange, yellow. Water-based paints are assumed
- Cerne relief outliner
- Brush – No 4 round short-handled craft brush
- Fine felt-tipped pen, water-soluble
- Scissors
- A4 sheet of paper
- HB pencil

Procedure

Wash and dry the wine bottle. Select three or four leaf designs from the pattern section of the book, and draw the shapes onto the bottle with a felt-tipped pen. If you wish to try different leaf layouts, the following procedure will help you with this.

Transfer the leaf patterns onto the sheet of paper.

Cut out each leaf profile and immerse in water; while the paper leaves are wet they can be placed on the bottle in the desired position. Try different compositions until you are satisfied with a design. Dry the bottle with a towel, taking care not to move the paper leaves. Just holding the towel against the bottle will remove the water. Draw around each 'leaf' with the felt-tipped pen and remove the paper leaves. Leave the bottle to dry thoroughly; do not use a towel or you will remove the lines. A hairdryer could be used to speed up this process.

Now that the bottle is dry, outliner can be applied. Lie the bottle down on a table or flat surface. Only a small portion of the bottle should be worked on at one time as the outliner will get smudged on the table if the bottle is turned. Alternatively, supports could be placed under each end of the bottle, preventing the area being worked on from coming into contact with the table. Apply the outliner along the inside of the felt-tipped pen line; try not to get any on the line as the liner will not adhere properly. Complete a portion and leave to dry for about 20 minutes.

When applying the glass paint, proceed in the same manner as with the outliner. Work on the level top part of the bottle, leave that to dry before rotating the bottle to paint other parts. Autumn leaves can best be painted by starting with the lightest colour, yellow, and adding a small amount of darker colour while it is still wet. Touch a little of the darker colour to the outer edges of the leaf and let the colours run together. As the bottle is curved, the colour will run on its own. Do not overbrush but let the paint mix naturally.

When you are satisfied with the colours (remember that the colours can be intensified or changed) leave to dry completely overnight. The next day you can carefully remove the felt-tipped pen markings with cold water.

Please note that the glass paint is not dishwasher proof.

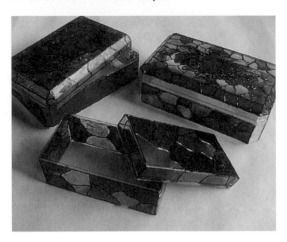

Project 3
Art Nouveau trinket box

Creating an Art Nouveau trinket box. This project requires a purchased glass box or an empty plastic chocolate box.

Materials required:
- Glass or plastic box
- Glass paint – pink, deep blue, night blue, emerald. Water-based paint assumed
- Palette
- Cerne relief outliner
- Brush – No 4 round short-handled craft brush
- Paper, or tracing paper A4 size
- HB pencil

Procedure

A simple Tiffany style design could be used for the box if you do not wish to use the Art Nouveau design.

Cut three pieces of paper for the pattern, one to fit the inside lid and the other two to fit the smaller and larger sides. One piece only is required if the box is square. Transfer the design onto the individual pieces of paper from the Art Nouveau design in the pattern section. Adjust the proportions to fit the dimensions of each piece of paper. Tracing paper is good to use when adjusting the design as it can be moved and the design followed underneath.

If you are using a plastic box with a removable lid, tape the paper design to the inside of the lid. Outline the design on the outside of the box with the cerne outliner. Place it to one side when finished. If the lid is hinged, follow the same procedure, but allow it to dry before starting another side. Tape the smaller design to the inside of the box on the appropriate side. Stand the box on its side so that outliner can be applied, allow to dry. Remove this design and affix it to the opposite end of the box. Apply outliner. The remaining sides of the box are completed in the same manner, using the larger design. When the outline has been completed, leave to dry. Do remember that the edges will also need to have an outline.

Start by preparing the pink paint for the flower on the lid, checking the consistency first before applying in the usual manner. Apply green to the leaves. The background can be completed using the two blues. Put the lid aside to dry. Finish all of the design on each side of the box and allow it to dry before turning it. Complete the other three sides in the same manner.

The colours shown are only a suggestion, try other combinations. Primary colours plus a neutral will give many colour possibilities. Check the colour mixing information in chapter 1.

If you are assisting other people, do let them be part of the colour selection process.

Silk painting

The process of painting on silk is very similar to glass painting. No artistic skills are required when creating a freestyle design.

Silk is stretched on a frame and held in place with special three-pointed pins or stenter pins. By keeping the silk wet while applying the paints or dyes, the colours will intermix and blend without

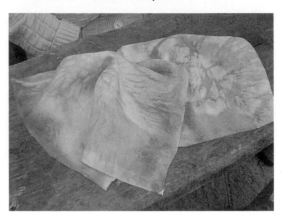

any hard edges, giving wonderful and startling effects. Much like the wet-in-wet process of water-colour painting, overprinting and layering other colours will add more depth to the design.

There is a large selection of water-based colours available for silk painting, both as paints and dyes. Paints need to be iron-fixed, while dyes are steam-fixed. Fixing the completed silk painting makes it washable and colour-fast.

As with glass painting, a design can be created and formed with an outliner or resist (gutta). Gutta is available as spirit or water-based in jars or tubes. Spirit-based gutta is removed with white spirits or by dry-cleaning whereas water-based gutta can be removed by washing after the silk painting has been fixed. Outliner is available in metallic and plain colours as well as pearlized. When fixed with a heated iron it remains in the silk.

As with all other projects throughout this book, I have suggested that water-based products be used. They are easily cleaned up and are not toxic.

When painting a particular design, you first create it on paper using a soft pencil or black felt-tipped pen. The design is then attached to the underside of the frame. Gutta is applied to the silk, following the outline of the drawing beneath. If using gutta from a tube a constant pressure and movement has to be used, in much the same way as outlining for glass painting. When the gutta is dry, paint can then be applied. As the gutta forms a barrier, the paint will be kept within the boundaries drawn by the gutta. Care must be taken when using water-based gutta, as it will stain if painted over; paint just up to the edge of the line. Be aware that as the gutta is water based, it will tend to break down if the silk is saturated with paint or water for any length of time.

There are several accessories available for silk painting including gutta nibs. These are metal spouts that can be applied to the nozzles of bottles or tubes. They are used to give a particular thickness of gutta line.

There are a number of silks available, each of which responds differently to paints or dyes. They all have a dressing that has to be removed by washing in hot soapy water.

A frame can be made or purchased; adjustable frames are useful as they can be used for many applications.

The following projects are simple enough, and without too much financial outlay give the reader a sample of the beautiful effects that can be achieved with silk painting.

Project 4
Painting on damp silk

This project will give the reader the opportunity to experiment with different colours, and create a free-flowing design. Salt crystals will be added to create starburst effects. With this type of silk painting large and uninhibited brush strokes are required. A larger silk painting can then be attempted, knowing that you will have good results with minimal materials and experience.

Materials required:
- Silk paints – water-based, vermilion, cerulean blue, yellow
- Palette, or three pattern-free, white china saucers
- Silk

- Three-point pins
- Gutta
- Wooden frame
- Brush – No 6 round, short-handled
- Water pot
- Natural sponge

Procedure

Prepare the silk by washing in hot soapy water and rinsing to remove the dressing. Cut the silk so that it is as large as the outside dimension of the frame. Lay the silk on the frame, pinning the centre of each edge to the frame and pulling it taut as you pin. Pin out to the corners along one edge at about 65 mm ($2\frac{1}{2}$ in). Start pinning its opposite edge, pulling the silk taut as you pin. Complete the other edges in the same manner. When working on a large piece, start by pinning each edge at its centre. Pin out towards the corners at about 65 mm ($2\frac{1}{2}$ in). But this time, pin only three or four pins from the centre in either direction. Pin the opposite edge in the same manner, pulling the silk tight. Again pin only three or four pins from the centre. Begin pinning from the centre along the third edge, using the same number of pins as you did for the first two edges. Proceed to pin the fourth edge, pulling the silk tight. Return to the first edge and continue the pinning process out to the corners. The silk should be stretched as evenly and as taut as possible.

I have successfully stretched very large panels using this method; it gives an evenly stretched surface on which to work.

To prevent paint from staining the frame, apply a line of gutta around the periphery of the silk. Allow it to dry; a hairdryer can be used to speed up this process. It will also be helpful to use the hairdryer to stop the natural spreading process of the paint.

Pour a little of each colour into the palette or saucers. The paint will dry somewhat lighter, you can check the colour as it will appear when dry by first testing it on a scrap of silk.

When applying paint to the silk in a freestyle wet-in-wet technique, start with the lightest colour and work towards the darkest.

Moisten the sponge and squeeze out most of the water. Tilt the frame and moisten the silk, starting from the top edge and working down. Wipe the sponge from left to right, completely and evenly moistening the whole piece of silk. Re-stretch the silk if necessary. While the silk is still wet, apply the yellow paint to a good portion of the surface. Next add a colour of your choice; it will blend with the yellow changing it to green or orange, depending on your chosen colour. When applying paint in this fashion, use the brush fully loaded and paint with sweeping brush strokes; do not dab at the silk or use timid strokes. Do not cover the yellow completely; it is important to leave some of the lightest colour showing. You might like to experiment with figure 'S' strokes, or angular lines. The 'S' stroke will give a softer, gentler appearance to the design, while the angular line will give a more dramatic feeling. To create a further dramatic effect, sprinkle table or pickling salt onto the silk while the paint is still damp. The granules of salt absorb the colour giving an attractive starburst effect. When the paint is dry, brush off all traces of the salt. It can now be fixed by ironing. Turn the silk to the reverse side and iron at the cotton setting. As the gutta penetrates the silk, use a thin cloth over the silk to prevent it from sticking to the base of the iron.

The edges of the silk can be finished by rolling them in and securing with small stitches placed about 10 mm ($\frac{3}{8}$ in) apart. Silk scarves and ties can be purchased with the edges pre-rolled. They can be stretched on a frame using small dressmaking pins, or better still, stenter pins. The latter have three small hooks that catch the rolled edges.

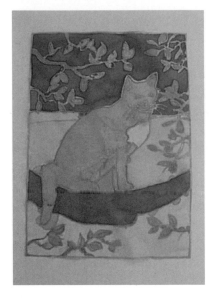

Figure 7.2

Project 5
Silk picture for framing

Creating a silk picture suitable for framing (Figure 7.2). One of the charms of silk painting is its versatility. Not only can it be used as a clothing accessory but it is also an excellent medium for creating unusual and interesting pictures. The following project gives step-by-step instructions for producing a picture suitable for framing. Unlike the last project, the paint will be applied on dry silk.

Materials required:
- Silk paints – water-based, vermilion, cerulean blue, yellow
- China saucers, three plain white
- Silk
- Three-point pins
- Gutta resist, silver
- Brushes – No 3 and No 6 round, short-handled
- Water pot
- Wooden frame

Procedure

Wash and stretch the silk as explained in the last project. Re-size the design to fit your silk piece, and place it directly under the silk. Attach it with tape or support it with a book that fits inside the frame so that it does not move. Carefully follow the outline with gutta. Remember to finish with a line of gutta completely around the design to form a frame. Check and fix any breaks in the outline.

Allow the gutta to dry completely. Pour a little blue silk paint into a dish. If you feel that the colour is too intense add some water. Test the colour on a piece of scrap silk before applying it to the working piece. Fill the largest brush and apply the paint to the sky area. The paint will spread to the boundaries made by the gutta. Take care not to flood it too much as the paint will run over the outline of the design. Keep applying the paint, making sure that any small corners are not missed. Paint fairly rapidly, as you do not want the wash to dry out. When the sky is completed allow it to air-dry. Leave any unused blue paint in the saucer; it will be used later.

Pour some yellow silk paint in another saucer, dilute if necessary. Paint the fields as indicated. Leave to dry. If you have some yellow paint left in the dish, add a little red to make a pale orange. This can be applied to the cat form.

In the saucer you used for the blue paint, mix a little yellow with the blue until you get a green you are happy with. Fill in all the leaves using the small brush.

To make a grey/brown for the tree branch, mix the complementary colours together – that is, blue and orange or red and green.

When the painting is completely dry, the water-based paint recommended for this project can be fixed with an iron. Please remember that silk dyes have to be iron-fixed. Remove the silk from the frame. Protect the ironing board cover with a piece of cloth, lay the silk right side down on the board. As it is possible that the hot iron will pick up gutta, lay another piece of cloth on top of the silk. Iron the silk with the iron set to the cotton setting.

A simple method of framing the completed work is to mount the silk in a clip frame. If you intend to use this method, select a frame size first and draw the design so that it will fit the clip frame. Make the design so that when the silk painting is completed, it can be cut a little smaller than the frame. This will create a border when the silk is assembled in the frame. If it does not fit proportionally adjust the design where necessary.

Cut off the excess edges of silk to the gutta outline. Dismantle the frame and clean both sides of the glass thoroughly. Place a piece of paper on the backing board and centre the silk on top of the paper. The glass can now be placed on top of the silk. Check for any marks on the glass or particles that may be trapped between the glass and silk. Re-attach the clips.

Chapter 8

Projects for festive and seasonal occasions

Winter/spring
Valentine's Day
Easter
Summer
Autumn
Christmas

I have found it really helpful, working in a residential home as I do, to create visual indications of the seasons and festivals of the year. Working on such projects stimulates interesting discussions among the members of the activities group.

The following projects are ideal for creating a festive or seasonal atmosphere, whether it is for a small area, a room, a feature wall or just a noticeboard. The completed items could also be used to decorate a child's bedroom or nursery.

As the month of January can be a little uninspiring, especially after all the festivities of Christmas and the New Year, time would be well spent working on projects for spring. The first project in this chapter, making paper daffodils, will bring some enjoyable spring colour into dull days.

Winter/spring

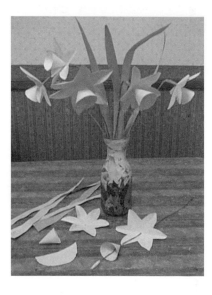

Making paper daffodils.

Materials required:
- Thin card, A4 size (three blossoms can be cut from one sheet)
- Acrylic paint, green, yellow
- Brush
- Water pot
- Pencils 2B, 2H
- Tracing paper
- Carbon paper
- Pencil compass
- Thick wire
- Green florist's tape
- Scissors
- Masking tape

Procedure

For three blossoms paint two sheets of the card on both sides, using the yellow paint. Allow them to dry.

Refer to the daffodil layout in the pattern section at the end of the book. Attach a piece of tracing paper over the design and carefully trace the design, using the 2B pencil. Remove the tracing paper. Attach the tracing paper, at one edge only, to the yellow card with masking tape. Slip the carbon paper under the tracing paper and press the design through using the 2H pencil. If you wish to make several daffodils, I suggest you make a template of the design by transferring it onto thick card. Carefully cut out the shapes of the flower petals. The template can be simply traced around to give the flower shapes. I found that many activity group members were able to do this task. Some were even able to cut out the shapes.

When the daffodil petals have been cut, fold each blossom petal to petal, three times. This will give you the centre and a little shape to the blossom. A small centre hole can be made with the point of the compass at this time.

To make the inside cone of the daffodil, set the compass to 55 mm ($2\frac{1}{4}$ in) and describe a circle. Cut out the circle of card making the edge serrated as you cut; use pinking scissors if you have them. Fold the circle in half, open it up and cut in half along the fold. Shape it into a cone, apply glue along the overlap and apply pressure until bonded.

The stem is made by cutting a piece of wire about 400 mm (16 in) long, twist two lengths together if the wire is very thin. Wrap about 50 mm (2 in) of the masking tape around itself at one end of the wire. Paint it yellow as this will represent the stamen. Push the wire through the cone and the centre of the petals. Put a dab of glue on the point of the cone and continue pushing the wire through until the cone is seated in the centre of the petal form. The tape should prevent the wire from going completely through. Using the florist's tape, wrap it several times around the wire stem at the back of the petals. This should effectively hold the stamen, cone and petals together. Wrap the rest of the wire with florist's tape. To make the daffodil leaves paint a sheet of card green on both sides. Allow it to dry. Cut thin strips 20 mm ($\frac{3}{4}$ in). Taper one end to a point, and fold in half along the entire length. Several more daffodils and leaves can be made to give a pleasant vase arrangement.

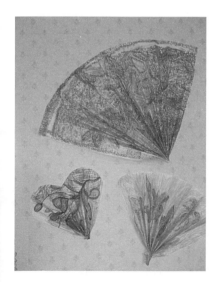

Project 2
Paper fans

Making paper fans. Paper fans can brighten up a room very quickly and will add a cheerful note on a grey winter's day.

Material required:
- Paper, A4 size
- Felt-tipped pen set
- Masking tape

Procedure

Outline flower and leaf shapes on the paper, or ask the person to draw a design of his or her own. By sketching out something first, no matter how simple, it will give those with little or no drawing skills a starting point for their colouring. Let the person select four or five colours, preferably not greys or browns. Start with the lightest colour and build up to the darkest and brightest. Felt-tipped pens are transparent to some degree so colours can be mixed by overlaying one colour on the next. It is always interesting to watch a colouring piece evolve. I will inevitably be asked what colour should be applied next. Usually I then ask the participants what colour they like and I might suggest something if things are going astray. If a piece is starting to look dull and uninteresting, I would suggest using complementary colours together to brighten the design.

Sometimes the people colouring will feel they have finished a piece but there is still a lot of white paper left. I encourage them to fill in all the white area, especially if the background has been left untouched. I suggest that they try using small strokes or dots using several different colours. (See shading techniques in chapter 1.)

When the colouring has been completed, start concertina folding, using 20-mm ($\frac{3}{4}$-in) folds along the shortest side of the paper. With the paper completely folded, tape or staple the folds together at one end. Colour the tape if necessary. Fan out the paper and attach it to the wall with a temporary adhesive compound such as 'Blu-Tack'. Several fans can be made like this giving a very colourful display. Fans made from larger paper can be cut into a curve at the top to give variety. You might also try folding a sheet in half along the longest side. By cutting a large curve at one end, and then concertina folding, the fan will open up to a heart shape. Which leads us nicely on to the next project.

Valentine's Day card

Project 3
Valentine pop-up card

Materials required:
- White card, A4 size
- Felt-tipped pen set of colours
- Pencil
- Ruler
- Scissors
- Craft knife
- Dinner knife
- PVA glue

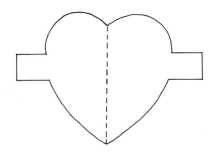

Procedure

Cut the card in half along the longest side, using the knife and ruler. Fold the longest side in half. If using thick card, score along this fold line with the back of the dinner knife; this will give a neater fold. Open the card and lie it flat. Working on the inside of the card measure out either side of the centre fold a distance of 45 mm (1¾ in) and make a pencil mark. They should be in the approximate centre of the panels.

Referring to the heart design, transfer the heart shape onto the other piece of the card. Cut out the shape and colour it bright red but do not colour the tabs. Fold the heart in half and fold back the tabs. Open the heart and apply a spot of PVA glue on the tabs; this should be on the same side of the card that was coloured. The heart should be a set in place a little above the centre of the card. Carefully align the bend of the tabs with the pencil marks, and press firmly. The card can be folded to hold the heart in place while the glue dries. The front of the card may be decorated with hearts if you wish.

€aster

Project 4
Egg mobiles

Materials required:
- Heavy white card
- Coloured felt-tipped pencils
- Pencil, 2B
- White thread
- Needle
- Scissors

Procedure

Draw and cut out one large and three small egg shapes. Cut out the shapes, and pencil in a design. As the mobile will turn both sides of the egg need to be coloured. Figure 8.1 gives some indication as to decorative designs, but many variations can be used. Colour both sides to your own liking.

The three small egg shapes can now be attached to the larger one by using three different lengths of thread. This will make them hang at different levels. To make them hang more interestingly, do not attach the thread in the centre, but towards either end. The shapes will then hang at an angle. A more complex mobile can be made by using a coat hanger or two bamboo canes tied in the centre to form a cross. More shapes can be added to this form of hanging arrangement. Make sure that the shapes do not get

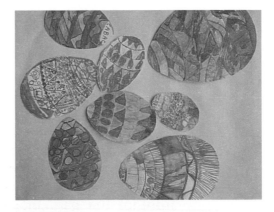

Figure 8.1

tangled up with one another. Check the balance before fixing in place.

Instead of colouring the mobiles, they could be decoupaged using Easter motifs cut from old Easter cards. Refer to chapter 3 for the decoupage procedure. Sweet papers, crumpled tissue paper and small pieces of material could also be used to decorate the egg shapes. Use a PVA glue to make sure that the pieces adhere properly.

Project 5
Easter chicks and mobile

An Easter chick mobile, using pom-poms, is easily made from yellow wool scraps.

Materials required:
- Wool
- Card
- Felt-tipped pen, blue
- PVA glue
- Darning needle
- White thread
- Scissors

Procedure

Cut two identical circles, from the card, about 75 mm (3 in) in diameter. Cut out a circle, about 25 mm (1 in) from the centre of each. So you now have two doughnuts. Thread the wool on the darning needle and pass it through the centre holes of the two cards held together. Keep on wrapping the doughnut with wool until it is thick all the way around. Snip the wool around the edges of the cards. Open the two cards enough to get a piece of yarn tied around the centre of the wool bunch. Tie securely and gently ease the two cards off the wool. Trim the ends of the wool as necessary to make an even pom-pom.

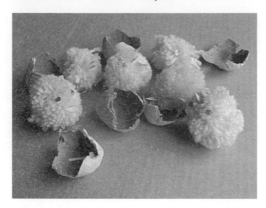

Figure 8.2

Several pom-poms can be made in this fashion. They could be of varying sizes by changing the size of the card circles. Try other colours too, it will make the mobile all the more interesting.

Cut out two beaks, eyes, and feet from the card; colour them on both sides and attach them to the pom-pom with a dab of PVA glue (see Figure 8.2).

The 'chicks' can be hung individually or attached to a hanging frame as described in the previous project.

Project 6
Chicks in a nest

Chicks in a nest make an excellent table centre piece or decoration for Easter. The process entails making egg shells with papier-mâché and chicks from the previous project.

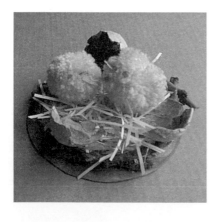

Materials required:
- Heavy card
- Shredded paper or yellow tissue paper
- PVA glue
- Plasticine
- Newspaper or paper towel
- Large dish
- Scissors
- Petroleum jelly
- Two chicks (as made in the previous project)

- Small household brush
- Egg cups, two
- Plastic film
- Craft knife
- Paint, water-based, colours white, brown

Procedure

Tear up the paper into small squares of about 15 mm ($\frac{1}{2}$ in). Prepare the glue by diluting it with water.

The egg shells are made by first making an egg form with Plasticine. Shape the Plasticine into an actual large size egg. Make two forms and cover with petroleum jelly. Lay pieces of the torn paper directly on the forms to completely cover each one. The process of laying and pasting pieces on the forms will get a little messy, so place the Plasticine forms in egg cups, then you will be able to apply paper without having to hold them. Lining the egg cups with plastic will make removal of the 'eggs' easier. Continue layering the egg forms with paper until you have applied four or five layers. You will find it easier to lay dry paper pieces on the egg forms, and then brush on the glue.

Take the forms out of the egg cups to allow the papier-mâché to dry thoroughly. When dry, paint them to resemble the colour of eggs.

After the paint has dried, cut into the papier-mâché at about the halfway point. The cuts you make need to resemble, to some degree, a broken egg shell from which a chick has emerged. Sharp angular cuts are preferable. After completely cutting around the form, carefully remove the papier-mâché shell. Depending on the paper used to construct the egg, you may have to paint the inside of the shell as well. Remove any traces of petroleum jelly first with warm water.

To make the nest, cut a 150 mm (6 in) diameter circle out of the card. This size can be adjusted to your own preference. Glue the shredded paper or tissue paper to the cardboard. Be aware that the colour of the tissue will run if too much glue is applied. The shells and chicks can be placed as required.

Project 7
Easter bonnets

Colouring is enjoyed so much by older people that I have included it in the bonnet decoration. I have purposely chosen white card stock for the construction, as it shows off the coloured designs much better. However, you may prefer to use more three-dimensional decorations, on a coloured card, and not have any hand-coloured design.

Materials required:
- Card stock: white, or colours of your choice
- Felt-tipped pen set
- Crepe paper – colours red, yellow, pink, green
- Pencil, 2B
- Scissors
- PVA glue
- Household brush, small
- Green florist's tape

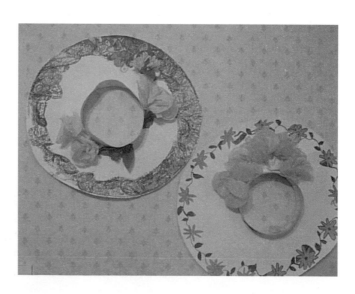

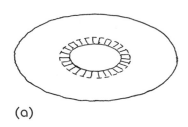

(a)

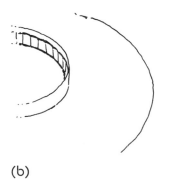

(b)

Figure 8.3

Procedure

Cut a circle from the card; this will depend on the size of brim you want. I use the largest I can get out of a full sheet of card, but your preference may be different. Start the hat by making the brim. First, measure the head of the person who will be wearing the hat. I use a piece of wool to measure the head size. Lay the wool in a circle in the middle of the card and draw around it. A smaller circle now needs to be drawn inside this inner circle, to make the opening. This should be an inch or so smaller all around than the wool, so that the tabs can be formed (see Figure 8.3). Cut around the inner circle to make the opening. Form tabs by making many small cuts at about 10-mm ($\frac{3}{8}$-in) intervals from the edge of the opening to the circle of the head measurement, Check to see if it will fit the person and adjust it if necessary. At this stage I draw out a design on the card to be coloured or I give it to the person to make up something to their liking.

There is a lovely 90-year-old woman who attends the activity sessions on a regular basis. She loves to draw flowers and is quite capable of drawing and colouring them without any help from me. Others need an outline to go by, but I do not influence their colour scheme, unless it is really necessary.

Cut a band of card 40 mm ($1\frac{1}{2}$ in) wide and long enough to fit the circumference of the circle of tabs with an inch overlap. Apply undiluted PVA glue to the tabs to give a good bond; affix them to the inside of the band (see Figure 8.3a). Make sure they are attached firmly; a little pressure may be required. Glue the overlap of the hat-band to itself.

The hat can be left and decorated at this stage or, if you wish, a cap can be added. Cut 25-mm (1-in) wide strips from card – they should be long enough to go over the top of a person's head – and attach to the band. The correct length will have to be found by measuring this distance while the hat is being worn. The number of strips will depend upon how you wish the cap to be finished.

I suggest that paper flowers be attached, along with some light fabric or netting.

While the hat is drying the paper flowers can be constructed.

There are many different and exotic papers now available for flower construction. Traditionally, crepe or tissue paper is used. It is readily available from art shops or from the suppliers mentioned in the reference section.

As the colours run when wet, the paper can be moistened to give an even more natural look to the flowers. Two different colours of paper may be dampened and squeezed together. The colours will run, making the darker colours lighter and streaked, and light colours will become tinted with darker ones.

Paper flowers are attached to and supported by the brim, therefore the petals and leaves can be made with tissue paper. However, tissue paper will give you a less rigid flower and leaf, which cannot be shaped too well. I recommend that crepe paper be used, as it allows the petals and leaves to be curled and formed to give a more natural look. Purchase crepe paper that is packed in folded rolls – 500 mm × 2500 mm ($19\frac{1}{2}$ in × 98 in). Stems can be made with wire covered with green crepe paper or florist's tape.

Project 8
Hat decoration, carnations

Materials required:
- Crepe paper, red and pink
- Scissors
- Rule
- Fine and thick wire
- Wire cutters or pliers
- Green florist's tape
- Masking tape

Procedure

To make eight pink and eight red carnations, cut two strips from the red and pink crepe paper, 60 mm

($2\frac{3}{8}$ in) wide. Along one edge of the folded crepe paper, cut sawtooth V's; pinking shears could be used if you have them. Unravel the paper and fold into four equal parts, cut at the folds so that you now have four pieces of equal length.

Hold one end of the paper – this will be the flower's centre. Start to concertina up the strip of paper in 10-mm ($\frac{3}{8}$-in) folds. Rotate the paper as you concertina. Make the folds looser as you get closer to the end of the paper. This will ensure that the carnation's outer petals are fuller and more open. If you choose to include a stem, insert the thick wire into the uncut end and secure by wrapping fine wire firmly around the flower's base. Cover about 30 mm ($1\frac{1}{4}$ in) of the flower base with the green tape and continue to cover the stem.

Carnation leaves could also be made and inserted at this stage, holding them in place with the tape. Cover the wire completely with the tape. Pull the outer layers of paper down to form the shape of a carnation and adjust the other layers as required.

Continue making the rest of the carnations and attach to the hat brim with spots of undiluted PVA glue.

Project 9
Hat decoration, roses

Materials required:
- Crepe paper, red, white, green
- Scissors
- Rule
- Thick wire
- Wire cutters or pliers
- Green florist's tape
- Rubber gloves
- Saucer
- Knitting needle
- Masking tape
- PVA glue

Procedure

Rose petals look more natural with variegated or streaked crepe paper. The procedure for this is as follows. Cut three sections of red and one piece of white crepe paper, 75 mm (3 in) wide from the still folded crepe paper. Put a little water in the saucer. With the paper still folded and wearing rubber gloves, dip one end of the red paper in the saucer of water. The water will be drawn up in the paper and start breaking the colour down. Gently squeeze the water out of the paper. Leave to dry before opening the paper out. The paper can be put into a slightly warm oven to speed up the drying process.

The white crepe paper can be streaked or variegated with the red using the following procedure. Place a cut piece (still folded) of red paper either side of the white. Dip the three pieces into a saucer of water; the water will be drawn up. To dampen the crepe paper further, lay each piece (still folded) on a piece of plastic or if near a sink, the draining board, and apply more water with a nail brush in the direction of the grain. As the paper is very fragile at this stage apply with very light brush strokes. Hold one of the folded pieces of red paper either side of the white and gently press together. The white paper will absorb some of the red pigment. Squeeze more of the water out, separate the three pieces and lay flat to dry. They could be put into a slightly warm oven to speed up the drying process. When the paper is dry, cut three scallops (see Figure 8.4). Unravel the crepe paper carefully. Fold the full length into three equal pieces and cut at the folds. You will now have three separate lengths, which will make three roses. For two larger roses shape two scallops and cut the full length of crepe paper in half. As the crepe paper is very wrinkly when unfolded, smooth out the paper between your thumb and fingers.

Curl each scallop (petal) by rolling the paper over a knitting needle. Make sure that the curls are all arranged in the same direction. Decide which end you wish to be the centre of the rose. If one end is

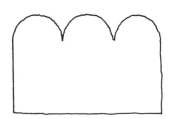

Figure 8.4

darker than the other use that end as the centre. Start rolling it up, with the curls facing out, so that the centre of the rose will be fairly tight. Once you've rolled the paper a few times, hold the base of the rose and start to pleat the paper, rotating the rose as you do so. As the paper is gathered, the petal shapes will be formed. By smoothing the petal ends further between your thumb and finger, you can shape the petals to a more natural appearance. Make the pleats a little larger as you get closer to the end of the length of crepe paper. This will open up the outer petals of the rose to give a more natural look. If you are going to include a stem, a thick piece of wire can now be inserted. Wrap a piece of masking tape around the base of the rose and the stem. A five-pointed calyx can be made from the green crepe paper; cut a piece 110 mm × 75 mm ($4\frac{1}{8}$ in × 3 in). Concertina the shortest side into five equal folds, press the folded paper as flat as possible. With the paper still folded cut it into a spear for about a third of its length. Unravel and attach to the base of the rose with a spot of glue. Wrap florist's tape around the calyx and stem. Adjust the petals if necessary.

Attach the flowers to the hat brim with a few spots of PVA glue. Leaves can now be shaped from the green crepe paper and attached to the hat.

Project 10
Hat decoration, paper daisies

Materials required:
- Crepe paper, yellow or white
- Scissors
- Ruler
- Pencil, 2B
- Masking tape
- PVA glue
- Florist's tape

Procedure

Begin the daisy construction by making the centres for as many daisies as you are going to make. Scrunch up half a sheet of a standard paper tissue into a ball, as tightly as possible. Using a 100 mm × 100 mm (4 in × 4 in) piece of crepe paper place the ball in the centre of the square. Wrap the crepe paper tightly around the ball, twisting it to make a tail and secure with masking tape. The centre can be coloured with any dark colour; make the rest of the centres and set aside.

Cut from the folded pack of yellow crepe paper, a strip 75 mm (3 in) wide. Open the strip and fold in half lengthways three times. You should now have a folded piece 90 mm × 75 mm ($3\frac{1}{2}$ in × 3 in). Cut slits along the 90 mm ($3\frac{1}{2}$ in) edge at 5-mm ($\frac{1}{4}$-in) intervals to create the petals, the cuts can be curved if you wish (see Figure 8.5). Dab a spot of glue on the centrepiece, unravel the crepe paper and start winding it around the centre piece. Continue winding, keeping the bottom of the slit just below the centre ball. Secure with tape when completely wound on. Cover the masking tape with florist's tape for a better finish.

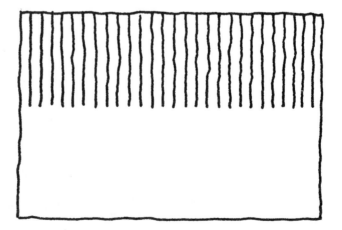

Figure 8.5

Summer

Summer months stimulate one to use intense and bright colours. The following project allows one to explore this to its utmost.

Project 11
Paper butterflies

Butterfly mobiles and wall decorations.

Materials required:
- White card
- Felt-tipped pen set
- Pencil 2B
- Glue stick
- 'Blu-Tack'
- White cotton thread
- Needle

Procedure

From the pattern section transfer the butterfly design onto the white card. Using the squaring-up method given in chapter 2, draw three sizes of butterflies, one large, another a little smaller and the third smaller still. Cut out the forms and use these as templates to create more butterflies if required.

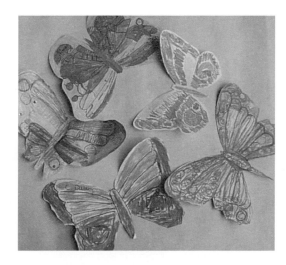

As with other projects that involve colouring a fairly large surface I break down the area into smaller segments. One could use reference material and draw actual designs of butterflies on the cutout blanks. I have shown this on my patterns, but they are not intended to be accurate.

Having laid out a design on the butterfly form, I pass it to a resident to be coloured. This is where it becomes interesting, as I give each person a totally free hand with colour schemes. They usually ask for suggestions, but I try to get them to choose colours of their liking. As both sides will be seen, they need to colour on the two sides. Feelers can be made with additional pieces of paper and glued in position.

The butterflies can be made either into a mobile or temporarily bonded to a wall or ceiling with 'Blu-Tack' or similar non-marking temporary adhesive. When making a mobile hang the largest first and hang the smaller ones from it. The butterflies will look more appealing if they appear to be flying. This can be done by tying a thread to both wing tips. It can then be pulled taut to set the wings at an angle to look like a butterfly in flight. Thread can be attached to this cross-thread and tied to another butterfly form. Attach other forms so that you have an interesting balance of three, five or seven butterflies.

Autumn

Project 12
Leaf rubbings

Leaf rubbings, mobiles and wall decorations.

Materials required:
- White copier paper, about six sheets
- White card
- Felt-tipped pen set
- Pencil 2B
- Coloured pencils or wax crayons, red, orange, brown

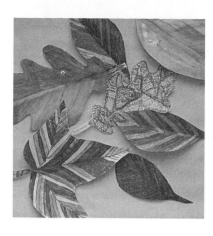

- Glue stick
- 'Blu-Tack'
- White cotton thread
- Needle
- Masking tape

Procedure

Gather as many different freshly fallen leaf shapes as you can find at this time of year. They will no doubt be a little wet so bring them indoors to dry. Before they start curling and losing their shape, lay each one on a flat surface. Place a piece of paper over one of the leaves. With a coloured pencil, gently rub the area of paper with the leaf underneath. The leaf veins will start to appear on the paper. Choose another leaf and do the same with this. A unique picture can be made by rubbing a variety of leaf shapes and sizes onto the same sheet. Build up the picture with the leaves set at various angles. By using different coloured pencils you can also create a more interesting design.

Leaf rubbings can be cut out to replicate the actual leaf. When a selection has been cut, it can be arranged to make an interesting autumn display. The paper leaves alone will not be stiff enough to be made into mobiles, but they could be glued onto card and hung as explained in the construction of a butterfly mobile.

Another use for the leaves when glued to the card is as a template. This, along with paper and felt-tipped pens, can be given to a person to create their own unique leaf colouring.

Transfer the leaf's profile to another piece of paper by tracing around its edge with a pen. Remove the template and draw lines to represent the veins. The leaf can be coloured with felt-tipped pens in whatever colour scheme is desired – it does not have to be the leaf's natural colour. A mobile can also be made if the profile is transferred onto card instead of paper.

The templates made from the leaves can be used in other applications throughout the book. Keep them in a file for future use.

Christmas

There are hundreds of different types of Christmas decorations that can be purchased, and more seem to appear each year. On the whole though I think nothing can beat those that have been produced by hand. They may not look as slick or have the latest jazzy style, but I feel that they have a certain quality and charm of their very own.

I have spent many hours with the residents, measuring, cutting and pasting together strings of paper chains. They all seem to enjoy it immensely.

Project 13
Paper chains

Materials required:
- Coloured paper, several different colours
- Ruler
- Glue stick
- Scissors

Procedure

If coloured paper is not available, plain paper can be coloured with watercolour washes, or felt-tipped pens. If you wish to use watercolours they can be applied with the paper wet, using the wet-in-wet technique described in chapter 1. This will give the completed paper chains an interesting and unique colouring.

Measure and cut strips of paper 230 mm × 25 mm (9 in × 1 in). Stand the cut pieces end on in a large pot so that the strips are accessible. If using a variety of coloured papers, a particular colour can then be easily selected.

Glue the strips into chains, making sure that they are well bonded, by pressing the glued portion firmly together.

Project 14
Mobiles

As with paper chains, the residents have made mobiles very successfully. I usually do the design work, creating an interesting shape for them to colour. Felt-tipped pens are their favourite medium, but watercolours or poster paint will work equally as well.

I make one large motif and two or three others of different sizes to be hung from it; this is explained under the Easter mobile project in this chapter.

I have found that the use of sequins has an extraordinary effect on a mobile. As the motifs rotate with natural air circulation, light catches the faceted sequins making them sparkle and shimmer. This really adds to the ambience at Christmas time, especially as many of these mobiles hang in one area of the room.

Materials required:
- Thick cardboard, preferably white
- Pencil, 2B
- Felt-tipped pens set
- Scissors
- Sequins
- PVA glue
- Saucers, two required
- Brush, small, as used for watercolours
- Cotton thread, white
- Needle
- Nail
- Hammer

Procedure

Select and enlarge a Christmas mobile design from the pattern section at the end of the book to fill approximately half an A4 sheet. Redraw the same design, or select another motif, reducing the size as necessary. If felt-tipped pens are to be used for the colouring, and the person is unsure where to apply the colour, draw lines on the forms as indicated. This again breaks down the area and gives the person a starting point. The lines do not have to be strictly adhered to, and it is better if they are not, as this will give the finished piece a truly original look. Both sides will have to be coloured but the second side can be completely different from the first. When all the forms are coloured, sequins can be applied.

The application of the sequins is a little tedious but well worth the effort. Put a good quantity of sequins in one of the saucers, in the other put a fairly large blob of undiluted glue. With the brush, apply a spot of glue where you wish a sequin to be affixed. With the same brush pick up a sequin, as there is glue left on the brush the sequin sticks to the brush quite easily. Transfer it to the glue spot. With the tip of the brush handle press down on the sequin so that it adheres firmly. Do not worry if the sequin is ob-literated by the glue; the glue will dry transparent and not affect the sparkle of the sequin. This process can be made easier with two people, one applying the glue, and the other setting the sequins in place.

How many sequins should you use? This is a matter of individual taste. If the bird forms are used, a sequin to depict the bird's eyes is striking enough I feel. But your taste may be quite different.

When the sequins have been glued to one side, let them dry thoroughly before turning the form over. Any wet glue residue will stick the form firmly to the working surface.

When both sides are completed, a hole should be made to take the thread where indicated. Before attaching the thread, lay out the various forms on a flat surface in their desired positions for the completed mobile. Make sure that they will not catch on one another or get caught on a thread. Once you have decided on the position of each piece, attach them to one another with thread. Hang at eye level near a radiator.

Project 15
Tissue paper stars

Paper stars made from tissue paper make an attractive Christmas window display. The stars are made up from several pieces of folded tissue paper; it is very important that all the pieces are cut exactly the same size. The folding is also somewhat intricate, so care should be taken with the cutting and folding. As the tissue paper is transparent any incorrect folds will show up badly when the star is hung.

Materials required:
- Tissue paper, light colours are preferable
- Ruler
- Pencil, 2B
- Dinner knife
- Glue stick
- Adhesive tape

Procedure

Tissue paper is difficult to cut with scissors, so I suggest that you fold it, and slit it with the knife. It is important not to use a knife with a serrated edge, as you will end up with a ragged cut. Fold the paper and make the crease as sharp as possible using the dinner knife. Cut the tissue paper by holding the folded edge down with the palm of one hand. Place the folded paper so that the fold is along the edge of a table. The knife can now be used to slit the paper along the crease. Do not try to fold and cut too many pieces at once.

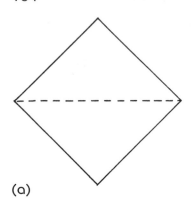

(a)

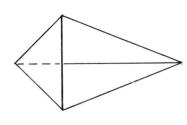

(b)

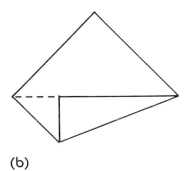

(c)

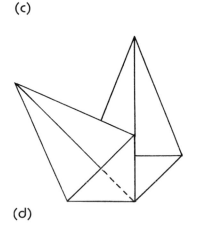

(d)

Figure 8.6

Cut a piece of tissue paper so that it measures 200 mm × 400 mm (8 in × 16 in). Fold and cut so that you end up with eight 100-mm (4-in) squares. Referring to Figure 8.6 make the points of the star. Fold a square in half diagonally, corner to corner. Unfold it and lay it in front of you with the crease mark running crossways (Figure 8.6a). The paper should appear diamond shaped. Take the corner closest to you and fold it so the bottom right edge of the diamond lines up with the centre crease (Figure 8.6b). Do this with the opposite corner, so that you now have what looks like a paper dart (Figure 8.6c). Fold the remaining seven pieces in the same manner. Make the folds nice and sharp by running the back of the knife along the crease. Using the dry glue stick, secure the flaps. A small dab of glue only is required.

Assemble the star by gluing each point together, overlapping as shown (Figure 8.6d).

The completed star can now be hung in a window with adhesive tape (see Figure 8.7). Small squares of double-sided tape placed at the points will be less conspicuous and ensure minimal damage to the star when removed from the window.

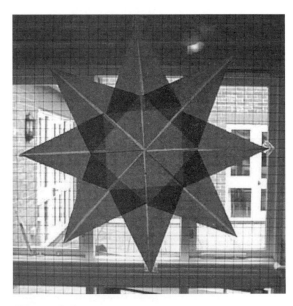

Figure 8.7

There are many other star-shape possibilities that you can try. Because the paper is transparent, the folds play an important part in the star's appearance when held against a light source. A small additional fold to the previous construction will give a different looking star with 16 points. Fold 16 squares as previously and include an extra fold to make the dart shape narrower. Try making a star with an oblong shape instead of a square and create some other folding patterns. As you will now be aware, lighter colours of tissue paper are preferable because of their transparent quality. When held against a light source, interesting patterns and various densities of colour will be seen; this is governed by the number and pattern of folds used.

Project 16
A paper angel

Materials required:
- White card
- Compass
- Craft or scalpel knife
- Steel ruler
- Pencil, 2B, 2H
- Tracing paper
- Coloured felt-tipped pens (optional)
- Cutting board

From the pattern section, transfer the angel design to a sheet of tracing paper. If you are making it a different size, the proportions should be kept similar to those on the pattern. Press the lines through onto the white card. As the design is symmetrical, the tracing paper can be simply turned over and the lines pressed through. This process is described in the construction of daffodils. Any light or unclear lines should be darkened.

Once transferred, cut along all the lines. Cut the detail and centre circles before cutting the outer circle. You will find a scalpel knife preferable to a

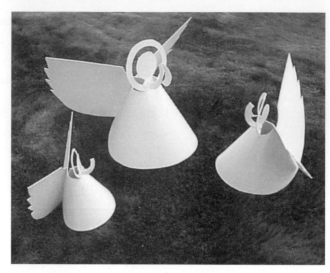

Figure 8.8

craft knife; moving the card and not the knife will give a better edge.

Colouring the angel is optional, but if desired, it should be done at this stage. As suggested in previous projects, guidelines could be drawn to indicate placement of colours.

The angel can now be formed by hooking the slits into one another (see Figure 8.8). Several angels of different sizes grouped together with a little holly make an attractive Christmas arrangement. The angels also make wonderful mobiles for a child's room, or over a baby's cot.

Pressing flowers and plants

Pressed flowers and leaves make wonderful material from which to make cards for special occasions such as Christmas, Easter, birthdays, etc.

Flowers that are to be used should be pressed carefully. A heavy book can be used but may not give the best results. A flower press, made or purchased, is by far the best equipment for this purpose. Flowers should be picked for pressing at their prime. The flowers should be completely dry, not wilting, and without any blemishes or tears. If the flower is at all damp it will create mildew in the press. If there is moisture, remove it by cutting the flower with a little of its stem. Put it in water so that it does not wilt, and keep it in a warm place, such as an airing cupboard. If you intend to press leaves, mosses, seeds, etc., they must be completely dry first.

When preparing material for the press, thick or bulky items such as rosebuds and trumpet flowers should be split in half. Place the cut side down in the press. Stems and calyxes should be removed. The delicate petals when pressed will then not have any unsightly marks. Spray flowers and small blossoms can be pressed all together, or alternatively with the petals and leaves separated to be reassembled when making the collage.

Making a simple press

A simple press can be made from thick plywood about 300 mm (12 in) square; two or three bricks can be laid on top of the loaded press to give the required pressure. An improvement on this would be to drill holes in the corners and insert bolts and wing nuts. This will give you the opportunity to make fine adjustments to the pressure and the press will be easy to move. To store the flowers in the press you will need several sheets of corrugated cardboard, newspaper and blotting paper.

To make a portable press, for use on walks, you will need two strong rubber bands, two pieces of plywood, a few sheets of corrugated cardboard and white blotting paper. The cardboard and blotting paper should be cut to the same size as the plywood.

If you intend to pick wild flowers be sure that they are not a protected species. A list of protected plants is available from the Department of Environment.

Care should be taken when loading the press. First, lay the outer board on a level surface; put a piece of corrugated cardboard on this followed by a few sheets of newspaper. Place a sheet of blotting paper on the newspaper. The items to be pressed are then laid on the blotting paper. Leave plenty of space between them as they will flatten and take up more room once the press is tightened. Be careful not to disturb the arranged items and add another sheet of blotting paper followed by several sheets of newspaper, then a sheet of corrugated cardboard. Layer another series in the same manner. Do not press flowers directly on newspaper, as the printing ink will transfer to the flowers. Continue layering until you have no more than six layers. It is a good idea to label each layer or keep a record of the items being pressed. Indicate what the items are and when they were placed in the press. When selecting items for each layer, keep them of a similar thickness. This is especially important for the bulkier ones, so that everything is pressed evenly.

Place the outer piece of plywood in position and secure. The press should be put in a dry environment, such as an airing cupboard. Drying will take between six and eight weeks. Plant material should be crisp and dry when ready; if it is at all damp or limp it should be returned to the press. If you wish to speed up the drying time, remove the absorbent papers from the press after about the second day and replace with dry papers. Great care is required not to disturb the items too much when transferring them. Changing the press like this every few days will reduce the drying time considerably.

There is always plenty of plant material that can be pressed. If you do not have a garden full of flowers, there is much to find in the countryside and by the sea, such as wild flowers and plants, grasses, seed pods, leaves and seaweed, all of which will press nicely and contribute to make a very interesting and colourful collage. Other materials that can be considered for pressing are fruit and vegetables. These should be sliced thinly before arranging the pieces in the press. As there is a high water content in these items, I recommend you change the absorbent material on a daily basis.

Project 17
Making occasional cards

Occasional cards, using pressed flowers and leaves.

Materials required:
- Pressed flowers or plant material
- Card A4 size. Note, hand-made card and paper are available at craft suppliers and work extremely well with pressed plant matter
- PVA glue
- Small brush
- Tweezers
- Craft knife

Procedure

Start by folding the card in half; if using heavy card, score the back first along the fold line. Once folded it can then be reopened and laid flat for ease of assembly. From the dried material that is available, choose a colour scheme or theme. From your experience with the colour wheel you will know that complementary colours such as red and green, blue and orange, yellow and purple, will vibrate with one another giving a highly contrasting colour scheme. Colours adjacent to one another will give a harmonious and much softer colour scheme. Any green that you wish to include should be chosen carefully so that it does not dominate.

When assembling the plant material, start from the outside and work towards the centre of the composition, overlapping as you go. Always lay out the material before finally gluing everything in position, any adjustments can then be made to the composition.

Pressed arrangements are also ideal for framing. Arrangements should be framed under glass with a mount. The mount will effectively prevent anything from becoming damaged by keeping the material away from the glass.

Chapter 9

Games

I have had much success introducing games into my activities programme. Many men do not wish to be involved with art and craft work but they will usually participate in a game. One of the most popular of these is dominoes. I have found that a quiz will also draw much interest from the women as well as the men. A team game can be adapted from most games and I have outlined some possibilities in the following section.

Dominoes

I'm sure this game, or adaptations of it, is played in almost every country around the world. It is said to have originated in ancient China, and found its way to England in the late eighteenth century. Along with darts, it is considered to be one of the most popular pub games played today in Britain.

There are various games one can play with dominoes; the game I am most familiar with is called the 'block game,' so-called because you are able to block your opponents' moves. This calls for a good memory, as well as having the blocking pieces of course. Two or four people can play at one time. There are a few different adaptations of this game. I can't remember who taught me, but it was probably a relative during my childhood days. The numbers are made up from a series of inlaid circular pieces, usually of ivory, but many are made from plastic or a resin these days. Each domino face is divided into two sections. Each section has a number of dots between one and six. A double six is the highest number in a dominoes set.

The game I was taught goes as follows. The set of 28 dominoes, or cards as they are sometimes referred to, is placed numbers down on a smooth table. The pieces are shuffled by moving them around until they are well mixed. If four people are playing, each person takes five cards; if two, the players take seven each. The remaining cards are left as a 'pool' on the table. Players stand their cards in front of them so that the numbers cannot be seen by their opponents. Play commences by the person having a double six putting it face up on the table. If this card is not in a person's hand, then the one with a double five begins. If this is not available a double four starts the game and so on. Play usually runs in a clockwise direction, so the person to the left of the first player needs a card with a six on it. If he has a six, he places it against the double six. If the player cannot play a card, then he has to knock on the table and pick up a card from the pool of dominoes. Play continues to the next player, who plays a card that corresponds to the number on the table. Double cards are usually placed crossways to the line of the other cards. The game continues until one player has played all his cards.

Tournaments can be set up, with team members playing in singles or doubles games. They can each play a number of games to decide the winner.

There are several variations of dominoes games available; they are played much the same as the traditional game. Characters such as animals, birds or insects replace the traditional white dots. Identical shapes have to be matched to continue the play. I have used the traditional game, as well as matching shapes, very successfully with older people.

Table skittles

The game was originally played with nine wooden pins, and a ball suspended by a cord that was in turn attached to a post. The player would stand with the skittles in front of him and aim the ball to knock down as many skittles as possible. However, as in darts, the players had to finish with a particular number of points. In skittles it was usually 31 to win the game. The skill comes in trying to finish one's score at the exact number of 31.

I have adapted the game to suit the people with whom I work, so the rules we play by are a far cry from the original. However, we have lots of fun, and that's the main thing.

A table skittles game can be easily constructed and can involve older people right from the initial stages.

Project 1
Making a table skittles game

Materials required:
- Cardboard tubes, nine in total
- Thick card
- Pencil, 2B
- Masking tape
- Small pebbles
- Small ball
- String
- Broom handle (cut to 700 mm ($27\frac{1}{2}$ in))
- Plywood cut to 300 mm (12 in) square
- Wood screw PVA glue (optional)
- Dish (optional)
- Magazines (optional)
- Varnish (optional)
- Household brush
- Acrylic paint

Procedure

The cardboard tube centre of a paper towel roll will make two pins; they can be covered with paper as in decoupage, or just painted. As the pins need to be quite heavy, one end can be closed off and the tube half filled with small pebbles. The top should also be sealed off to prevent the stones falling out when the pin is knocked over. To seal the ends of the tube, stand a tube on a piece of thick card and describe a line around the circumference. Remove the tube and cut out the circle. Make 18 circular discs in this manner. They are attached to the tube with masking tape. Run the tape over the disc while it is in position at the end of the tube, and up the side of the tube for about 40 mm ($1\frac{1}{2}$ in). Another piece of tape is then wound around the tube to cover the tape and make a firm attachment. I would suggest that the tube is covered as a decoupage piece; that is, glue on small pieces of paper. When they are dry, several coats of varnish are applied, which will make the pin quite durable. More information on the decoupage process can be found in chapter 3.

In the original game, the pins are set in a 200-mm (8-in) square, with the point of the square facing the player. Because I have to adapt things a little, I write a number on each pin and set them up as in a bowling alley. Numbering the pins makes it quite challenging for the players who will go for the highest number. This makes them realise very quickly that more accuracy with their throw is required to get a good score.

A broom handle attached to a piece of square plywood will make a suitable post. Attach it with a screw from the underside. The screw should enter the post to a depth of at least 30 mm ($1\frac{1}{4}$ in). If a sturdier post support is required, use thicker plywood and attach the post to it with three angle brackets. The base may have to be held by another person, or a book or two could be placed on the base. This will help to prevent the post tipping over, in event of exuberant throws.

Placement of the post is quite crucial so that the ball can swing properly. It should be a little to the left and forward of the pins. You can either purchase a small ball, or make one as I did by winding wool around a small stone until it is the size of a golf ball. Adjust the weight if necessary, by adding more wool. My reason for making a ball from wool is that my players get rather erratic with their throws and even manage to hit a few spectators. So a soft woolly ball was the answer.

Table skittles is a lot of fun with our group. Everyone gets involved, whether they are playing or not. It could easily be played as a tournament on a weekly basis.

Memory games

One aspect my art training, which was more years ago than I care to remember, was to learn to draw from memory. To improve my ability to do this, a number of objects were put before me – actually there were quite a number. I had to study them for a few minutes, walking around to observe all relevant detail. A cloth was then placed to cover all the items. Then came the tricky bit: I had to draw as many items as I could remember, with as much detail as possible, that were now hidden under the cloth. I found that now, many years later, I still look at objects with a more inquisitive bent than most people. Now back to the memory game.

The same approach can be taken to set up a game of memory. The players, instead of having to draw the objects, could write them down. A time limit should be set to make the game more challenging. To make this into a team game, the players could shout out the items as they remember them and a score be kept. Several rounds could be played, removing and adding different items.

Find the pair

This game is an old time favourite, especially with children, so there are many ready-made picture versions available at the toy counter. I remember playing it in my younger years with a deck of ordinary playing cards. However, as an activities project, I got the residents to make a set, getting those at a session to draw and colour, on heavy card, two identical objects. This sort of game is very useful to monitor a person's memory recall.

Put 'n take

This is an adaptation of a game that I played in my youth. Instead of the two brass spinners in my original game, I use a single spinner made from card.

Project 2
Constructing a put 'n take spinner

Materials required:
- Thick card
- Compass
- Craft knife
- Felt-tipped pens, red and green
- Pencil
- Metal ruler
- Wooden bamboo skewer
- Bradawl
- Masking tape

Procedure

To make the spinner set the compass to 55 mm ($2\frac{1}{4}$ in) and describe a circle on the card. Without altering the compass setting, set the point anywhere on the circle and describe a mark on the circle. Now set the point on this mark and describe another mark. Continue in this manner until you have six marks on the circle at equal distances.

Join all the points with straight lines, and cut along the lines to make a hexagon. Draw lines to connect the points to the centre. Number the segments from 1 to 6. Write 2, 4 and 6 in green and write

TAKE below each number. The other numbers should be in red; write PUT below them.

Cut the wooden skewer to 70 mm ($2\frac{3}{4}$ in). With the numbered side uppermost, make a hole in the centre of the hexagon. Push the sharp end of the skewer through to protrude about 20 mm ($\frac{3}{4}$ in). Wrap masking tape around the skewer, taping it tightly to both sides of the hexagon card. Holding the top of the centre post the spinner is started with a snap of the fingers. It will now spin like a top and will come to rest on one of the flat sides.

Two or more players are given 'chips' (safety matchsticks, buttons or whatever). Each player spins the spinner, and whoever spins the highest number starts the game. This player now spins the spinner and waits for it to stop. The directions are followed and the spinner is passed clockwise to the next player. The winner can be decided by the player having the most 'chips' after a certain time, or the person left after the other players have lost all their 'loot'!

Quizzes

Articles required:

- Flip chart or white board
- Pen (white board marker and eraser)
- Paper

One of the most popular quiz games I use in the home is an adaptation of a game called 'Tell me'. The game consists of several cards with simple questions on them, and a spinner with the alphabet. The spinner is spun, and it stops on a letter, say 'D.' A card is turned up and the question read out, such as, 'what is a place you would like to visit?' The answer has start with the letter D. The game continues until all the questions have been answered.

I usually have the residents organised into two teams. Because it is important for players and non-players alike to be involved as much as possible,

I have made an alphabet wheel, with an arrow as a spinner. I take this around to each person and get them to spin the arrow, whether they are players or not.

The points are marked on a large white board, so that everyone can see how their team is doing. A count is made at the halfway point, usually at teatime. At the end of the session a tally is made of all the points. A round of applause is given for the winning team and the runners up.

On each person's wrist is tied their team colour; this helps them remember which team they are in. It is also easy for me to decipher where the points should go. I let the players give as many answers as they can, but not the same answer more than once. In the case of identical answers being given at the same time, I give each person a point.

I play it as a weekly team tournament, between two teams of five players a side, or more if possible. Each week the scores are added to the preceding week's score. At the fourth week, the final tally is made and the winning team has their team colour attached to a trophy. It has proved to be a lot of fun and is much enjoyed by the residents.

Any number of questions can be made up, depending how long you wish the game to last. They can be simple or quite difficult depending on the group. The game can also be played individually with a small prize given to the person getting the highest number of correct answers.

Hangman/snowman word game

Articles required:

- Flip chart or white board and eraser
- Pen
- Paper

This game is one of first that I learnt to play as a small boy, probably everyone else did at around the same age as well. As I wanted to adapt the game for the residents as a team game, I use a snowman image rather than the usual hangman. It is a cheerier symbol, and when the snowman team wins, the last feature added is the mouth, which can then be a large smile. If you wish, you could choose to use a clown figure or any other figure for that matter, it just needs 13 details that have to be drawn.

This could be played as a weekly tournament just like the previous quiz. To play the game as a team game, select two teams and get them to sit a little distance from one another. The teams could choose a name for themselves to make it more interesting. Give a piece of paper and pencil to both teams and get each member to write down a word. Toss a coin to decide which team is to find the word, and which is to build a snowman; let us say the 'B' team is to find the word.

Decide which word the 'A' team wishes to start with and put a dash to represent each letter of that word on the board. The 'B' team now has to suggest letters that might be in the hidden word. If there is more than one of the same letter in the word and that letter is chosen, all the letters have to be written in. The game continues until the blank spaces are all filled. Points can be awarded for the number of letters in the word. Bonus points can be gained if any member of the 'B' team is able to guess the word before all the spaces are filled. I suggest five points plus the number of letters in the word. If they guess wrongly, five points go to the 'A' team. The game continues until the word is found, whereby the 'B' team receives all the points denoted by the number of letters in the word. If the snowman is completed first then the 'A' team receives the points. It is a good idea to have each member in turn suggest a letter as there are bound to be some that are more reluctant to speak up.

Another word can be selected and the same team can try to guess the new word or, alternatively, the roles could be reversed.

If you do not have enough players to make it into a

team game, I suggest the following. Get each person to write a word on a piece of paper; this, of course, should be done without anyone else seeing the word. If a person has difficulty thinking of a word, give them a book to look through. The person could even point to a word in the text. Make sure the person's name is also on the sheet. Collect all the sheets. Start the game by selecting a word from one of the sheets. Call out whose word it is, the rest of the group can now play against that person.

Twenty questions

Articles required:

- Paper
- Pencil

This is an old parlour game that was very popular in Victorian times. I remember that it was also a popular listening programme for our family, before the advent of TV, back in the good old wireless days. It can also be an enjoyable lounge game, played again with two teams, which we will call 'A' and 'B.' A toss of a coin decides which team has to think of an object. Let us say team 'B' thinks of an object, which should be written down. Team 'A' now has to try to find what the object is by asking questions, 20 being the maximum number that they can ask. Team members should again take it in turns to pose questions. Permissible answers to the question are either yes or no. To keep score, it is just a matter of a point being awarded to team 'B' for every 'No' answer. When the object has been successfully identified, or 20 questions have been asked, a new round commences; the 'A' team thinking of an object and the 'B' team having to ask the questions. Rounds can be alternated like this for, say, 10 rounds. The number of rounds can be as many as you wish, of course.

Picture puzzles

There are many jigsaw puzzles available to purchase either new or second hand from thrift shops or jumble sales. Older people certainly do enjoy hunting through the myriad of pieces trying to assemble what is sometimes a very complex picture. However, I have found that a simpler form of puzzle is required at times. By taking a familiar scene from a magazine, gluing it onto a heavy card, and then cutting it up into segments, a picture puzzle can be made very easily. There are many possibilities that one can try, from pictures of pets, flowers, ships, cars and trains, to an enlargement of a family photograph. The segments can be cut into large simple shapes, or small and intricate ones, depending on the level of difficulty required.

The final picture can either be mounted onto a piece of hardboard and hung or kept as a puzzle to be used again. It could also be made into a competitive game by having two teams with similar puzzles try to complete theirs in the fastest time.

Shove halfpenny

As a boy, I recall many enjoyable winters' evenings playing this game with my father and brother. This was a family interactive game, quite a while before the days of television. Since those days I have lost track of the whereabouts of the board, but I remember that it was made of slate. I think it would be a great game to revive, so I have included it in this chapter. I'm sure many older people will remember the game, as it was a very popular pub game and may still be today.

Ten lines are etched across the width of the board, making nine spaces, or 'beds,' as they are called. The game is played by two players with five halfpenny coins each. As these coins are no doubt hard to find I suggest the use of two-pence coins, or large washers. They should be smoothed down a little on one side, to make them slide easily. One set of coins is played heads up, the other tails up, to avoid any confusion. If washers are used, they should be marked in some way. To make the coins run easily, the surface of the board is dusted with french chalk or talcum powder.

A toss of a coin decides who will start. Play commences by a coin being placed on the board so that it overlaps the front edge. The coin is pushed sharply with the heel of the hand. All five coins have to be played before the other player tries with his coins. As all the coins are left on the board until the last has been played, it makes for skilful 'shoving' by the second person to get their coins in, and their opponents' coins out of the beds. The object is for either player to get three coins in each bed. The first to get three coins in each of the nine beds wins the game.

I have managed to track down the regulation board size, and will include it for those adventurous enough to make one. Although my board was made from slate, mahogany was also used, and I might suggest that counter-top material could be an alternative. This should be mounted on thick plywood or wood composition with a thin application of the proper glue. It is essential that the finished surface be absolutely flat. To prevent the board from moving when the coins are hit, secure a piece of wood on the underside of the board, below the front edge. This will act as a stop against the edge of the table on which the board is placed.

The board size is 610 mm long by 380 mm wide (24 in × 15 in) Ten lines are etched the full width of the board, 32 mm ($1\frac{1}{4}$ in) apart making nine spaces or 'beds' as they are called. At the playing end, the lines start 95 mm ($3\frac{3}{4}$ in) from the front edge and leave a space of 230 mm (9 in) at the farthest end. Any coins landing in these end areas are deemed out of play. Two more described lines run the full length of the board, 32 mm ($1\frac{1}{4}$ in) in from either side. This margin is where the score is kept by means of a chalk mark for each coin in the bed. A water-soluble felt-tipped marker could be used in place of the chalk, or strips of paper could be taped down each side. Lines could be drawn to correspond with the lines of the beds on the board. Coins landing in this area are out of play.

Scoring is not done until all 10 coins have been played. If any player scores more than the allowable three in one bed, the extra points go to the opposing player.

Group games – singing and music

I introduced music and party games to the residents and they responded surprisingly well. Their ability to remember lyrics to older songs was amazing, even the very confused and those with acute memory loss joined in the singing. Others, who did not sing, clapped their hands to the beat, and managed to hit a tambourine or shake a rattle, to some sort of regular beat. Some even got up to dance a little. I make it a point to include music in an activities session, even if it is just background music. If members of the group recognise a song and start to sing, I immediately take the opportunity to have a sing-along, even if it is just for a brief moment. Most really enjoy this addition to an activities session and join in heartily.

Festive occasions are an excellent time for activities to include music and party games. The games will, of course, depend on the mobility of the participants, but seated games such as pass the parcel, and toss the hoop, or those including a balloon, are the sort of games that I would suggest. I have also tried pin the donkey's tail, which proved to be great fun. For those who are not mobile, I take the donkey image, which is attached to a pin board, to the seated player. He or she can then be blindfolded, and attempt to pin the tail.

Musical balloons

As older people are not so quick on their feet, I use this adaptation as an alternative to musical chairs. Instead of the players jumping up and scrambling for a vacant chair, balloons are passed around instead. Participants sit in chairs, not armchairs, as they would be difficult to move. They should be facing one another and arranged in a circle. Just as in musical chairs, there is always one participant without a balloon. Music is started and the balloons are passed around. When the music stops, the person without a balloon is unfortunately out of the game. The person and the chair are removed from the circle. The chairs are repositioned in the circle, one balloon is removed and the music is restarted. This adaptation works well and is lots of fun. The game does require helpers, especially to help move people less mobile. It would be ideal as a game for those in wheelchairs.

Floor games

Floor games are ideal for groups in a lounge setting. The following games can be played from armchairs set in a circle.

Project 3
Roll a ball

Materials required:
- Three small balls
- Eight pieces of paper, about 200 mm (8 in) square
- Felt-tipped pen, variety of colours

Procedure

On the eight squares of paper write as large as possible, the numbers from 1 to 5. I omit the number six as it could be mistaken for a nine. Some numbers will be written twice. Set these in the centre of the circle. They can be close together or separated a little. Offer the three balls, one at a time to a member in the circle. They then have to throw the ball to land on a square of numbered paper. After the three balls have been thrown, the score is tallied and recorded. Another player then continues the game, and so on until all the players have had a turn. The highest number wins the round. If there is a tie, those players can then have a play off to decide the winner.

I found a set of soft filled juggling balls to be better than regular balls, as the balls wobble a bit and do not roll in a straight line. This makes the 'shot' much more unpredictable, making it possible for any person to try their luck without feeling they have to be an 'ace' lawn bowler.

Floor skittles

Another activity that has proved to be great fun in a group situation is floor skittles. For the more mobile, the skittles can be set up as in a bowling lane. For those not so active, it can be played from armchairs. Instead of the person bowling the ball at the skittles, a piece of PVC household guttering is used as a chute. As gravity is the only force to propel the ball, the skittles may have to be placed closer to the players. Skittles for this game can be made from the cardboard core of kitchen towels.

Project 4
Making a floor skittles game

Materials required:
- Paper towel roll
- Paper towel cores, nine required
- Thick cardboard
- Masking tape
- PVA glue
- Scissors
- Small pebbles
- Emulsion primer (optional)
- Household brush (optional)
- Acrylic paint (optional)
- PVC gutter, cut to about 110 cm (43 in)
- Three small balls

Procedure

Place the end of a paper towel core on the cardboard and describe 18 circles. Cut out the circles. Glue each circle to one end of each tube. To secure the end further, tape each one, running the tape across the end of the sealed end and up the side of the tube. Tape can be wrapped around the tube and over the tape to secure the end further. Once the pebbles have been placed in the tube for stability, the open ends can also be sealed in the same manner as the 'bases'.

As colour plays an important part in motivating people, I suggest that the tubes be coloured with bright colours. The tubes will have to be primed first as cardboard does not take paint well. The tubes can be made the same colour or a variety of colours. Instead of painting, decoupage could be used; the coating of varnish suggested for decoupage will make the tubes quite durable.

I suggest a method of scoring is by numbering the skittles; give each coloured skittle a number or simply paint numbers on the skittles.

Bowling

Another game that is immensely popular among the residents is a bowling game which I have adapted using a children's boules set of balls, the chute mentioned in the skittles game and an upturned cardboard box.

The flaps of the open end of the box are removed. A hole or holes are cut in the side of a cardboard box at the edge of the open end. The holes need to be a little larger than the balls. To strengthen the box at these crucial points cardboard braces are glued on the inside from the front to the back of the box. The box is placed, open end down, at one end of the room, preferably against a wall. The player sits in a chair at some distance from the box. This can be adjusted to suit the ability of the player. The chute is given to the player and adjusted to point at one of the holes. A ball is placed on the chute and released. No effort is required, since gravity and the weight of the ball send it on its way, hopefully to enter the hole in the box.

More often than not the ball misses the hole and hits the box; hence, the need for the strengthening braces.

One important aspect of the game is that, although only one player can 'bowl' at a time, the onlookers, including staff, become totally involved in the outcome of each delivery. Cheers and applause reign supreme when a ball finds its mark.

Play the music and dance

As important a part of the activity sessions as music is, there is another related activity that I highly recommend – a dancing event. Of course, such an activity involving physical movement is governed by the capabilities of the members in the group.

A dance is a good way to mark occasions such as the New Year, Valentine's Day, St Patrick's Day and so on.

One such enjoyable event was a Valentine's masked ball that I organised. The residents made hand-held masks during the weeks running up to the day. The masks were handed out at the dance and the music began. Strauss waltzes were played to evoke a Viennese mood. As the music played I invited the more mobile women members to dance. The positive response was, as always, very gratifying. Eyes sparkled at my request and soon I had a partner who began a few small steps, moving in time to the waltz music.

Games and a sing-along are good companions to dance. The variety of activity means everyone has an opportunity to become involved if they so wish.

Patterns

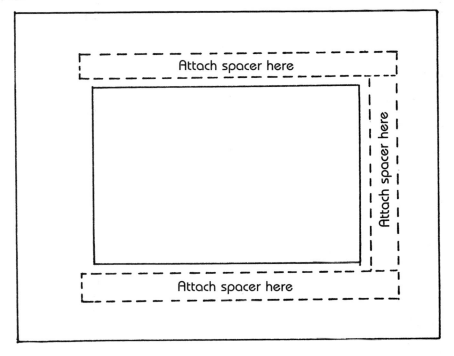

Attach spacer here

Attach spacer here

Attach spacer here

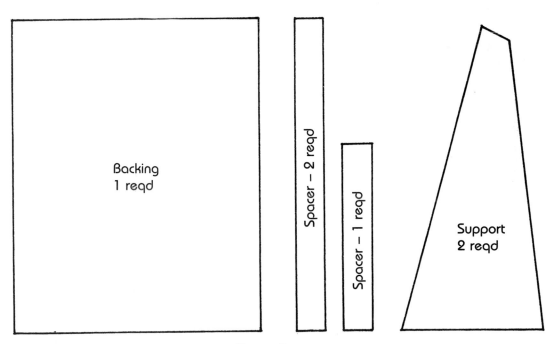

Backing
1 reqd

Spacer – 2 reqd

Spacer – 1 reqd

Support
2 reqd

Picture frame

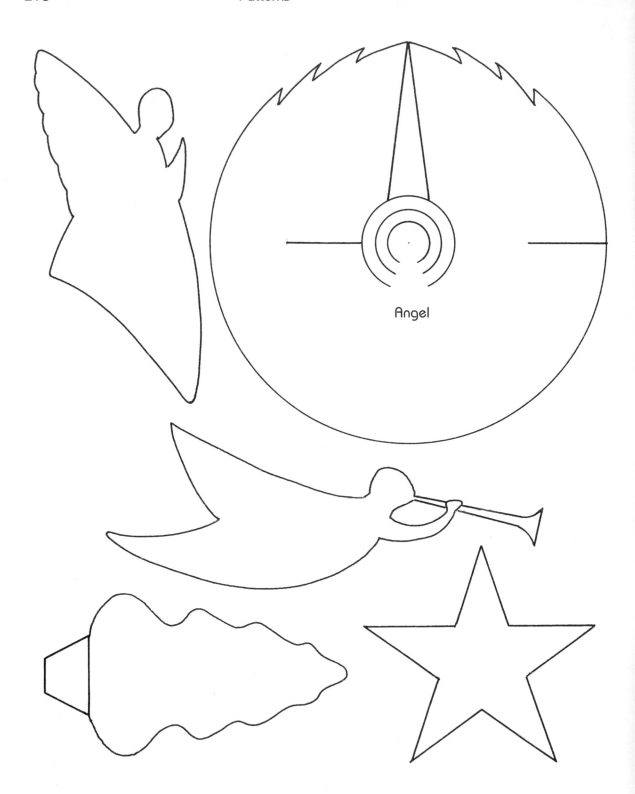

Angel

Rose petals

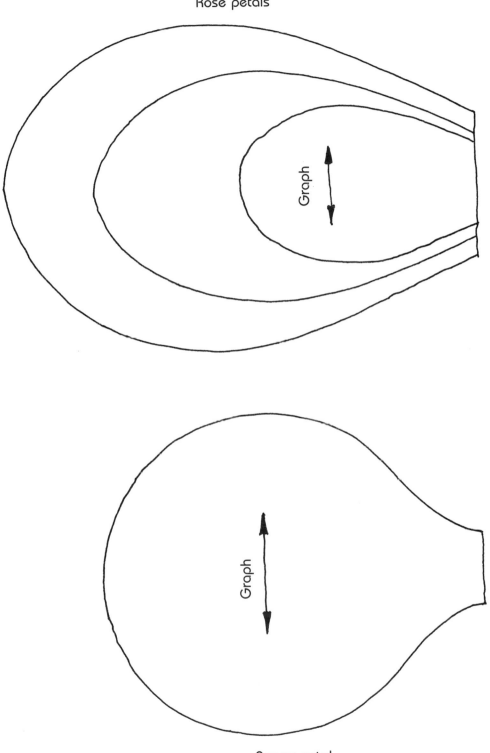

Graph

Graph

Poppy petal

Daffodil

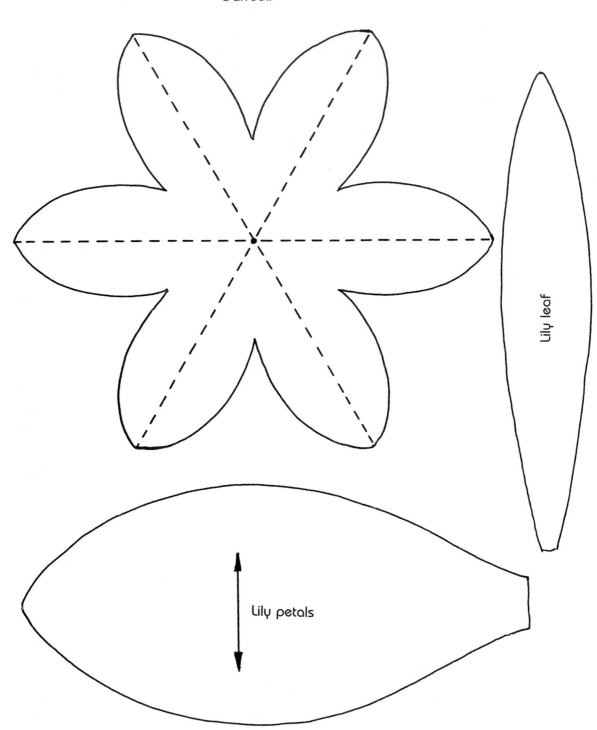

Lily leaf

Lily petals

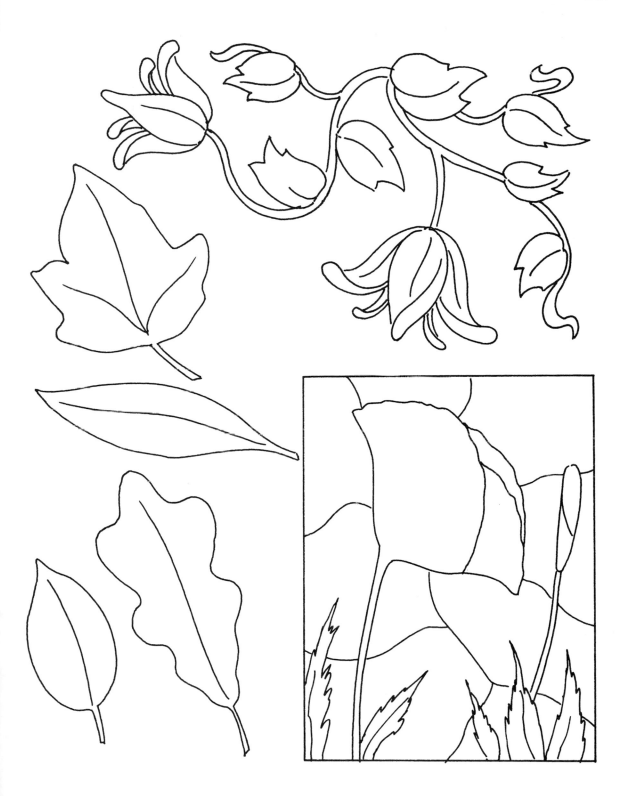

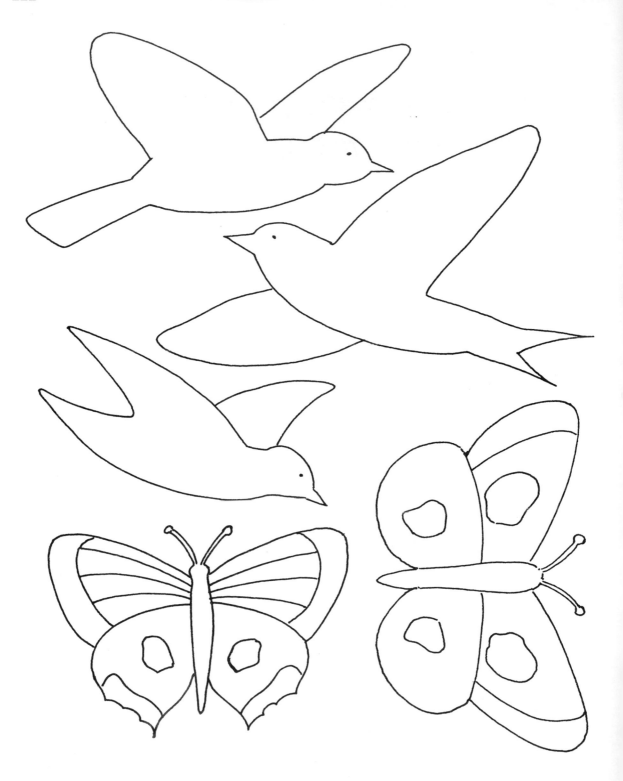

Useful addresses of suppliers of art and craft materials

Homecrafts Direct

PO Box 39
Leicester, UK
LE1 9BU
Tel: 0116 2513139
Fax: 0116 2514452
Email: speccrafts.co.uk

Mail order supplier of art and craft materials

Art Express

12–20 Westfields Road
Leeds
W. Yorks, UK
LS3 1DF
Tel: 0113 2436996
Fax: 0113 2436074

Mail order suppliers of art and craft materials

Craft Creations

Ingersoll House
Delamare Road
Cheshunt
Hertfordshire, UK
EN8 9HD
Tel: 01992 781900
Fax: 01992 634339

Mail order and showroom. Specialize in greeting card blanks and accessories.